The King of

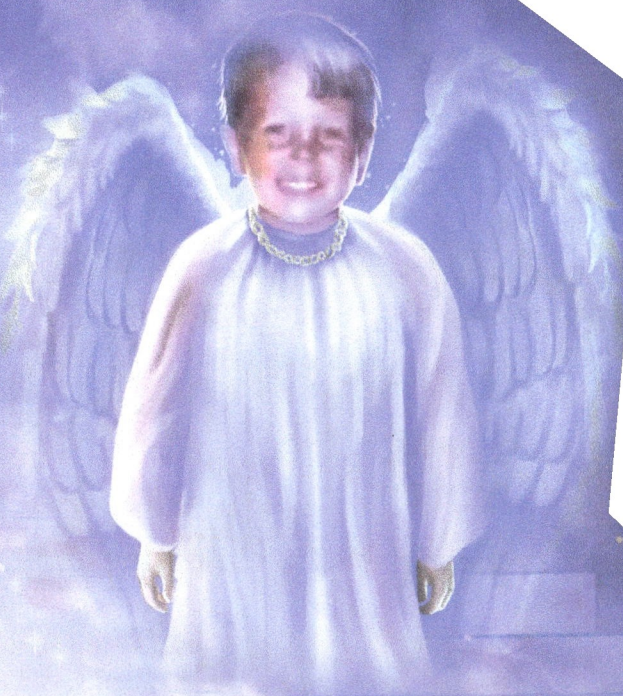

Mary L.

Joshua M.

When Angels Fly

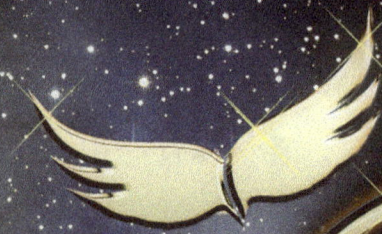

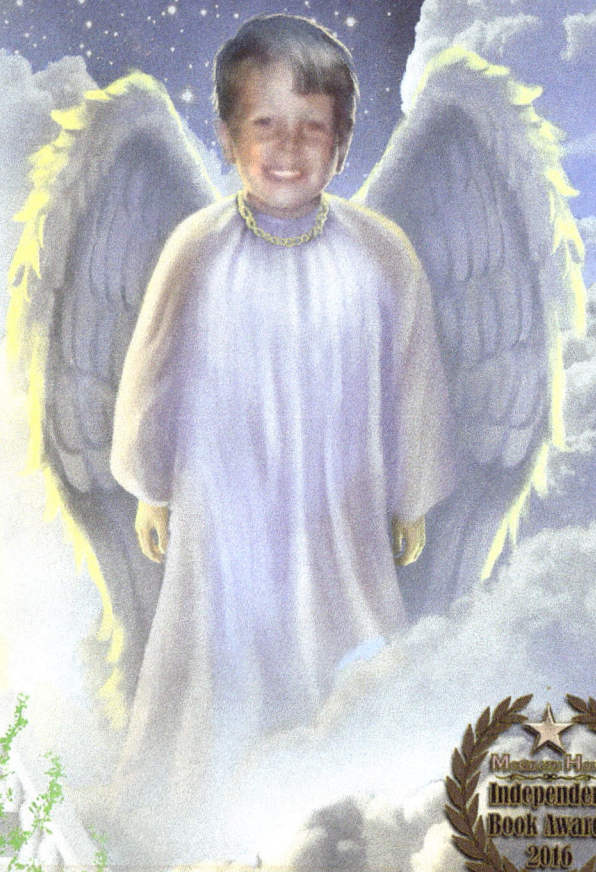

S. Jackson
A. Raymond

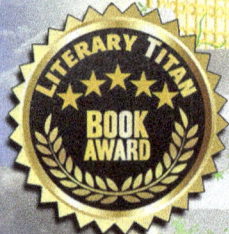

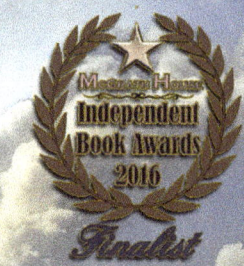

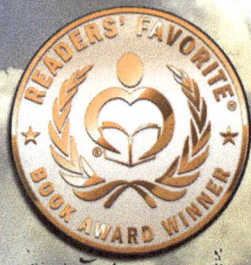

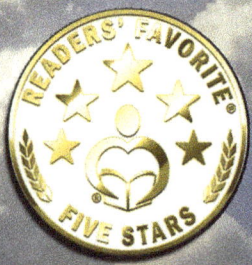

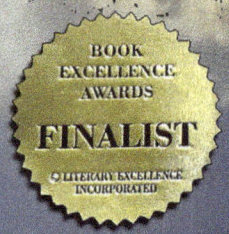

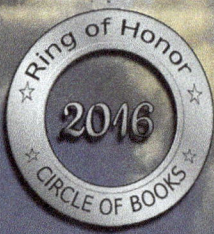

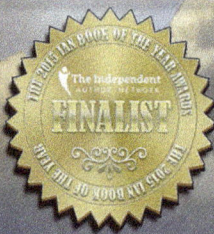

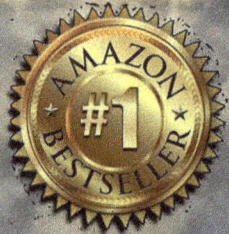

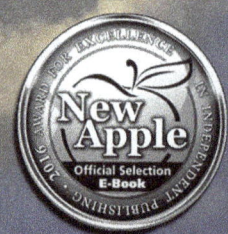

The King of Loss

Screenplay

By Mary L Schmidt & Joshua Vickery

Based on the book, When Angels Fly

By S. Jackson, A. Raymond, M. Schmidt, & G. D. Donley

Library of Congress Cataloguing-in-Publication Data

ISBN-13: 978-0-578-59358-6 (Mary L. Schmidt, Gene. D. Donley, M. Schmidt Productions)

ISBN-10: 978-1-0878-0908-3

Cover design by Mary L. Schmidt, S. Jackson, & A. Raymond

First edition published October 2019

https://whenangelsfly.net

Email: mary.mmschmidt@gmail.com

ARTISTIC STATEMENT

MARY SCHMIDT

The King of Loss didn't come from an idea. It isn't a dream I once had, nor is it the story of a relative, close friend or casual acquaintance. As a matter of fact, it isn't a story at all. It's my life.

It is a horrific and unimaginable thing to lose a child, but to lose two children is nearly incomprehensible for most. Not only did I have to lay to rest two of my children, but the second was my five-year-old son who lost his life while battling cancer. I can tell you with certainty that there is no other feeling of heartbreak so tremendous as when a mother, for months, has to helplessly watch as her child fights for his life.

Two decades removed from the tragedy, I was finally able to share my life's story; not because it gave me something to do, but that it might help others who have walked in my shoes.

Having kept a daily journal throughout my son's battle with cancer, I was able to revisit those painful memories and write them down in the book, *When Angels Fly*. However, after the overwhelming positive response that followed, I knew this would impact many more lives when shown on the big screen.

Therefore, having the book transcribed into a movie not only seemed like the right thing, but the ethical and perfect thing to do.

The King of Loss will surely not only minister to those whom have lost a child, but will also bring them the knowledge of the hope that awaits them at the end of this terribly dark journey.

THE KING OF LOSS: JOSHUA M. VICKERY & MARY SCHMIDT

SYNOPSIS

On her wedding day, set in the mid-80's in Silverthorne, Colorado, nineteen-year-old SARAH LOGAN makes a promise to God, that if he would grant her the gift of children, unlike her extremely abusive mother, ETHEL JACKSON, she would become a mother of whom he would be proud. How is Sarah to feel toward God, however, when she loses her first of three sons to a miscarriage, and God allows her youngest to fall ill with cancer at the age of four?

Based on real life events, after an entire childhood of suffering mental and physical abuse from her mother, Sarah dreams of one day escaping Ethel's vicious talons and running off to marital bliss with her Prince Charming. Her fairytale quickly turns horror story, however, when husband, HENRY LOGAN turns out to be an abusive, jealous, alcoholic husband.

Sarah needs someone whom she can love, who will also love her back. Her hope of having a joyous life with a fairytale ending is once again ignited when discovering that God has finally granted her the gift of a child.

Sarah's best friend since childhood, ANNA, 22, is a cute, little brunette. Raised as a tomboy, Anna works for her father's company as a Master Electrician; full of feistiness and the Spirit of God. Though Henry could care less about the pregnancy, Anna is with Sarah every step of the way.

When almost full-term with the baby, Sarah is pleasantly surprised one evening when Anna shows up at her front door with tons of baby gifts. It is the same evening when Sarah shares her concern with Anna that her baby hasn't been very active as of late. As most any friend would do, Anna nonchalantly tells her that all is well, and that Sarah should just pray to the Good Lord and let him take care of the rest. However, Sarah's world begins to cave in as she finds herself heading for an emergency checkup with her obstetrician the very next morning.

Faith, Hope and Love all hang in the balance for Sarah when she learns that her baby boy, Joshua, suffered death by strangulation of the umbilical cord. Though Anna tries to comfort Sarah, the damage has already been done. Sarah's bitterness toward God begins to protrude from the depths of her soul.

Due to her character and integrity, Sarah remains faithful to her abusive husband and moves forward with life. Like finding a burning ember of light amidst a bed of pitch-black coals, Sarah once again discovers hope for her fairytale ending, when she eventually has a son, NOAH, followed eighteen months later by her baby boy, ELI.

Over the next few years, Sarah takes great pride in raising her two sons, while at the same time attending school to become a Registered Nurse. Though she endures the beatings from Henry, she refuses to allow him to spew his fits of fury onto Noah and Eli.

One day in the heat of battle, after Henry leaves a cherry on Noah's cheek, Sarah locks herself in the bedroom with her two sons, protecting them from his rage. In the midst of it all, from out of nowhere little Eli asks his mother, "Who is Jesus?" Exhausted from years of abuse, pain and tragedy, embittered, Sarah tells him that Jesus is "no one," and that she will protect him and his older brother from now on.

Late that same night, with a little help from Anna and a huge Italian man, Sarah sneaks out of the house with her boys and heads to Durango, Colorado to begin a new life of peace and freedom, though she could have never prepared herself for the road that lay ahead.

Shortly after the move, Eli was diagnosed with having mononucleosis and sinusitis. As the weeks and months role by, Eli shows no improvement. To no avail, Sarah continues to battle with the doctors as to what is infecting her child, until one morning in February of 1990, she awakes to find one side of Eli's face is drooping.

Through weeks of more tests being run on Eli, and constant badgering from Ethel and Henry, Sarah discovers that her newly laid fairytale foundation is on the brink of collapse when hearing that Eli has a soft tissue mass – a pharyngeal tumor extending up through the cerebral fossa and into his brain cavity. Though in shock, Sarah's first inclination is to tell God that he's already taken one of her children, and to stay away from Eli.

Eli and Sarah spend the next several months at the University of Colorado Hospital. Though it breaks her heart to spend so much time away from Noah, Sarah is steadfast at Eli's side. After his chemo treatments, and a few final scans, things are looking up as Eli and Sarah are released to go home in mid-July of 1990. Shortly thereafter, however, Sarah receives the news that one of Eli's scans show remaining cancer in his lungs.

On July 31st, Back at the University of Colorado Hospital, Sarah is helping to prep an already frail Eli for lung surgery, when he asks her a question that would send chills through any loving parent: "Mommy, am I going to die?" In loving motherly fashion, Sarah does her best to comfort him, until she is completely taken back when Eli says, "I want to go to Heaven, Mom. I want to go to Heaven and Jesus."

Heartbroken to hear these words from her little boy, Sarah has enough bitterness towards God to respond by telling Eli that we don't always get what we want.

Over the next eight months, little Eli fights for his life, while Sarah fights the demons that stand between her and God. Though little Eli loses his life on October 15th, 1990, at 11:35pm, the autopsy reveals that he won his battle with cancer. There was none to be found within his tiny body.

In the end, Sarah makes her peace with God. Her final conclusion is that life isn't a fairytale, but a restless journey that we all must travel. However, no matter which road you choose, they will all lead you to the Land of Paradox. While there, you will find the best and worst that life has to offer. You will find both joy and pain, happiness and sorrow, love and hatred. Unlike Cinderella, it isn't a prince that Sarah finds in the Land of Paradox, rather, it is two kings. The One she calls her Lord and Savior, and the other... The King of Loss.

SUPERIMPOSE:

> "Are not all angels ministering
> spirits sent to serve those who
> will inherit salvation?"

HEBREWS 1:14

1   INT. JACKSON FAMILY KITCHEN- EVENING (1965)

A tiny, five-year-old Sarah Jackson sits all alone at a tiny
table, nervously staring down into the palms of her hands
that rest upon her lap.

From across the table, only remnants of her face can be seen
through flowing locks of golden hair.

The clanging of pans in the b.g. cause little Sarah to jump,
raising her head to stare aimlessly across the table through
her beautiful blue eyes.

Sarah's mother, ETHEL JACKSON (mid-30s) appears much older in
her grandma nightgown and house-shoes, stands over the
kitchen stove with her back to Sarah. Ethel shuffles across
the scarred linoleum floor to the kitchen sink, then back to
the stove; never turning around.

Sarah's bottom lip quivers as she bites down, hiding the
fear.

Ethel turns around. With saucepan in hand, a cigarette hangs
limp from her sly smirk. Sarah meets her mother's glare with
a hint of defiance, folding her arms across her chest.

An old, empty ceramic bowl with a clanking spoon slides
across the table, resting in front of Sarah. Sarah doesn't
flinch.

Green peas cascade from the saucepan, forming a miniature
green mountain in the bowl.

Staring ahead, Sarah refuses to acknowledge her dinner.

Ethel leans down within a hair's breadth of Sarah's ear...

                    ETHEL JACKSON
                 (gritting teeth)
             Eat your peas... now!

Defiantly, Sarah doesn't move.

3

<u>THE KING OF LOSS</u>

Written by

Joshua M. Vickery & Mary L. Schmidt

Based on the Memoir, "When Angels Fly"
By S. Jackson & A. Raymond

Mary Schmidt
P.O. Box 371
Ellsworth, KS 67439
785-472-8665

4

Tossing the pan on the table, Ethel grabs the spoon in one hand and squeezes the child's jaws with a tight grip between her thumb and fingers of the other, painfully prying open Sarah's mouth while shoveling in a spoonful of peas...

                    ETHEL JACKSON (CONT'D)
          I said eat, Sarah!

Sarah's resistance comes to an end, as Ethel continues to gorge her with massive amounts of peas. Crocodile tears roll down the toddler's cheeks.

                    YOUNG ADULT FEMALE (V.O.)
               (wistfully, sardonic)
          Peas. They are saturated with
          vitamins C, E and Zinc. Full of
          nutrition, right? Maybe if she'd
          looked at it that way, then she
          wouldn't have had so much
          resentment towards Ethel, her
          Mother. Maybe she *wouldn't* have
          felt as though she was being
          punished.

(O.C.) Ethel continues to force-feed little Sarah, as clumps of peas begin dropping onto the table.

                    YOUNG ADULT FEMALE (V.O. CONTINUED)
          But when peas are being served to
          you at almost every supper, and
          you're forced to finish every last
          bite, *every* time - which was always
          more than any five-year-old could
          possibly eat - then maybe you, too,
          could begin to understand that what
          Ethel was doing was not a
          manifestation of her love. (beat)
          She force-fed her peas... almost
          daily... to the point she would
          always, well...

2   INT. JACKSON FAMILY BATHROOM- NIGHT

Little Sarah hugging the toilet. Vomiting violently.

                    YOUNG ADULT FEMALE (V.O.)
          ...See her meal for a second time.

FLASH FORWARD:

3   INT. UNIVERSITY OF COLORADO HOSPITAL- NIGHT 1990

It's the young hands of a thirty-year-old woman. One hand
writes in a journal that rests in her lap, while the other
holds tightly to a Kleenex tissue. A wool sweater blankets
her arms down to the wrists.

There is one wadded tissue that rests alone at her side,
laying on what appears to be the seat of a pew.

                    YOUNG ADULT FEMALE (V.O.)
              When she was a child, she didn't
              know that evil mothers really
              existed. Cinderella had become her
              inspiration because of the
              hardships she had to endure from
              her stepmother. But her inspiration
              continued for little Sarah even
              into adulthood... along with
              Ethel's abuse. Therefore, she did
              what any abused nineteen year old
              would do... she ran. She ran right
              into the arms of Henry.

BACK TO SCENE:

4   EXT. LOGAN FARM AND HOMESTEAD- DAY

Sarah (19), in a sundress, and Henry Logan(25), wearing
cowboy boots, jeans and a western shirt, stand before a
drunken minister and a few of Henry's friends and relatives,
in a pasture at Henry's father's farm.

                    YOUNG ADULT FEMALE (V.O.)
              Oh sure, maybe he wasn't a prince
              of whom Cinderella would have
              swooned over, but Sarah didn't
              dismiss him. Though they had met in
              a smoky bar, she couldn't help but
              to think that he was the missing
              piece to her fairy-tale ending.

5   INT. JACKSON FAMILY LIVING ROOM- DAY

SLOW MOTION, Ethel is dragging nineteen-year-old Sarah
through the living room by the hair, followed by kicks to the
stomach and blows to the head.

>   YOUNG ADULT FEMALE (V.O.)
>   The truth, however, was that she
>   was willing to do anything to
>   escape the vicious talons of her
>   mother.

Sarah's step dad is trying to restrain Ethel.

>   YOUNG ADULT FEMALE (V.O.)
>   Due to the fact that her
>   stepfather, Paul, couldn't be there
>   to save her all the time, I suppose
>   Henry was the next best thing.

FLASH FORWARD:

6   INT. UNIVERSITY OF COLORADO HOSPITAL- NIGHT 1990

The young hand of a thirty-year-old woman continues to write
in a journal that rests in her lap.

>   YOUNG ADULT FEMALE (V.O.)
>   So thankful to finally be free from
>   her mother's wrath, on her wedding
>   day she made a promise to God: That
>   if He would grant her the gift of
>   children, then she wouldn't be like
>   Ethel... SHE WOULD BECOME A MOTHER
>   OF WHOM HE WOULD BE PROUD.

BACK TO SCENE:

7   INT. THE LOGAN'S FAMILY CABIN- DAY

SUPERIMPOSE:
               Silverthorne, Co. 1982

It's noon. HENRY LOGAN is just getting out of bed, still
dressed in last nights western-wear.

He stumbles into the bathroom to relieve himself of last
nights hangover.

While urinating, he hears SARAH talking to someone at the
front door. Finishing up, Henry makes his way down the narrow
hallway of the tiny home, rubbing the sleep from his eyes.

Sarah, dressed in scrubs, stands at the front door talking to
a man. She notices Henry has awaken...

                    SARAH
                (to the man)
            Well, thank you. You have a nice
            day as well.

Sarah nervously closes the front door.

                    HENRY
                (snarling)
            And just who the hell was that?

                    SARAH
            Uh... it was just the mailman.

She flashes the envelopes at Henry before placing them on a
tiny kitchen table.

He quickly makes his way toward her, jabbing his finger in
her face.

                    HENRY
            You don't ever talk to him! If he
            stops by again, you come get me.

Henry reaches down, grabbing the mail.

                    SARAH
            He was just delivering the bills,
            Henry.

Gripped tightly in his hand, Henry viciously turns and slaps
her across the face with the mail, knocking her to the floor.

                    HENRY
            I said come and get me, or I will
            kill you. And don't ever let me
            catch you talkin' to another man
            again. Do you hear me?

Sarah, fighting back the tears.

                    SARAH
            Would you please stop with your
            accusations!

Henry grabs her by the arms, picks her up, slams her against
the wall, pinning her with his body weight. The plaster
cracks behind her head.

Nose to Nose with Sarah...

                    HENRY
            You're mine, woman. No one else
            will have you.
                (MORE)

                              HENRY (CONT'D)
                    You're sealed to me in marriage.
                    Remember? No one can have you, but
                    me.

A single tear rolls down Sarah's cheek as anger flexes her
jawline.

Henry hurls her into another wall. She grunts as The impact
steals her breath.

Gasping for air, Sarah pleads with him.

                              SARAH
                    Please... Stop...

Like a place-kicker, Henry delivers a three-step drop kick to
Sarah's stomach.

                              HENRY
                    Stupid hag.

Sarah pretends to pass out after the blow to the ribs.

She lays in the floor, waiting for Henry to slide on his
cowboy boots and make his exit. As the front door slams
behind him, she gasps, finally able to take in a deep breath.

Using the battered wall to help climb to her feet, she limps
down the hallway.

8   BEDROOM

Retrieving a suitcase from beneath the bed, Sarah pulls open
a drawer and begins packing.

With trembling fingers, she zips up all she has left in her
life. She turns to find Henry standing in the doorway.

                              HENRY
                    What the hell do you think you're
                    doing? Did I say you could leave?

She freezes in fear.

Henry arrogantly, slowly struts toward her.

                              HENRY (CONT'D)
                    Don't you know that we're supposed
                    to be together forever? Or do you
                    not remember our vows... "Till
                    death do us part."

Sarah sits on the bed as he approaches, dropping her suitcase.

Henry raises her chin with one hand, caressing her face with the other.

> HENRY (CONT'D)
> You know what that means, right? It means I'll kill you before I ever let you leave me.

8   *SMACK!* comes the backhand, leaving her laid out in agony across the bed; sobbing.

9   INT. DOCTOR'S OFFICE- DAY

The day after her beating, SARAH sits upright on an examination table, wearing a patient's gown. DOCTOR #1 (60-ish) inspects her ears with an otoscope.

> DOCTOR #1
> (frustrated)
> You have a concussion, with two busted and bleeding eardrums, and you're telling me you've dropped the charges...?

> SARAH
> Well, I--

> DOCTOR #1
> Look, it's none of my business what you do with your life...

Removing his examination gloves.

> DOCTOR #1 (CONT'D)
> ...But I see this all the time, Sarah. It never ends well for anyone involved.

Sarah slowly steps down from the examination table.

> DOCTOR #1 (CONT'D)
> All I'm asking is that you reconsider your decision to drop the charges.

Sarah winces at a sharp pain in her side.

                         SARAH
          I appreciate your concern, but
          doesn't everyone deserve a second
          chance?

                         DOCTOR #1
          Young lady, you and I both know
          this isn't the first time you've
          visited my office.

Shaking his head in disbelief, he writes a prescription and
hands it to her.

                         DOCTOR #1 (CONT'D)
          This will help with the pain until
          your body manages to get healed up.
          And tell your boss down at the
          nursing home that *I* said you need a
          couple days rest.

Gently placing his hand upon her shoulder...

                         DOCTOR #1 (CONT'D)
          Sarah, your body isn't made to take
          this type of abuse... Just think
          about it.

10   INT. SILVERTHORNE COFFEE SHOP- DAY

SARAH sits alone at a tiny table, sipping on a hot cup. There
is another hot cup sitting across the table.

SARAH is alarmed when a tiny bell jingles as the entryway
door opens. It's ANNA (22), a petite and feisty tom-boyish
brunette, always with a sense of humor.

ANNA peaks back toward a corner booth, grimacing at the
strangers in "her" booth.

                         SARAH
          Anna, over here.

Anna spins left, approaches Sarah while keeping her gaze
fixed on the strangers in "her" back corner booth.

                         SARAH (CONT'D)
          Oh, chill out. It's not your coffee
          shop.

                         ANNA
          But it is my booth.

Anna's eyes brighten when spotting an awaiting cup o'joe.

                    ANNA (CONT'D)
          For me...?

                    SARAH
          No. It's for my other best friend.

                    ANNA
          Sorry I'm late. I was helping daddy
          wire a new residential.

                    SARAH
                 (chuckling)
          Who would have ever pegged you as a
          master electrician?

Anna takes a sip after settling in.

                    ANNA
          Ah. You're too good to me, Sarah.

                    SARAH
          I'll remember you said that.

Anna explodes at Sarah in frustration...

                    ANNA
          Are you kidding me?

Sarah's taken back at Anna's outburst. All eyes from other
coffee sippers are drawn to the disturbance.

Sarah leans in to quieten the tone.

                    SARAH
          Kidding you about what?

Anna scans the room to ensure their privacy.

                    ANNA
          The black dot on your cheekbone
          that you so poorly tried to hide
          beneath your Revlon.

                    SARAH
          Is it that noticeable?

                    ANNA
          Is it that...

Anna pauses, forcing herself to stay calm.

                    ANNA (CONT'D)
          Is it noticeable? Two years, Sarah.
          This has been going on for two
          years.

                    SARAH
          I just... I just want to be--

                    ANNA
          A mother, right? Yeah, I get it.
          But Sarah, there's plenty of guys
          out there who can help you with
          that.

Awkward silence. Sarah grins.

                    SARAH
          Did you just say that?

They both giggle.

                    ANNA
          Look, that came out wrong. But you
          know what I mean. You are young and
          beautiful, Sarah... inside and out.
          You deserve a good man. Spencer
          says that Matthew asks about you
          all the time.

                    SARAH
          Anna, your husband's best friend,
          Matthew is it, isn't the answer to
          my problems. And divorce is wrong
          anyway.

                    ANNA
          Not when it's like this.

Anna reaches across, taking Sarah by the hand.

                    ANNA (CONT'D)
          Look, you know I just love you,
          girl.

                    SARAH
          I know you do. And I'm so lucky to
          have a friend like you.

Anna relaxes back, taking a sip of coffee.

                    ANNA
               (facetiously)
          Well at least we can agree on
          something.

The two ladies chuckle.

11   INT. LOGAN'S FAMILY CABIN- DAY

SARAH stands by the living room window in her pajamas. In the dimly lit room, she tries to focus on a little, plastic strip in her hand.

                    SARAH
          Oh, C'mon.

She reaches, separating the window's curtains, allowing the early morning sunlight to kiss her slightly bruised cheek bone.

Closing her eyes, she inhales a deep breath. Smiling.

Refocusing, she quickly takes another glance at the plastic strip in her hand. Still nothing.

                    SARAH (CONT'D)
          You've got to be kidding me. C'mon
          already.

Childlike, she anxiously shuffles over and flops down on the couch. Nervously tapping her foot on the floor.

Closing her eyes tightly...

                    SARAH (CONT'D)
          ...Please God.

Raising the plastic strip, she takes another peek.

She places her free hand over her mouth as a tear streaks down her cheek.

12   Looking down, Sarah removes her hand from her mouth and places it gently over her tummy.

                    YOUNG ADULT FEMALE (V.O.)
          For two years she had been praying
          fervently for a baby; for someone
          whom she could finally love, who
          would also love her back. And by
          the Grace of God, He had finally
          breathed new life into her fairy-
          tale.

Sarah springs to her feet...

                    SARAH
               (screaming)
          Henry!

She jolts down the hallway toward the bedroom.

12   BEDROOM

SARAH leaps onto the bed next to a passed out, hung-over
HENRY.

                    SARAH
          Henry! Henry!

Startled, Henry tries to open his heavy, drunken eyes.

                    HENRY
          What the hell's goin' on?

                    SARAH
          Wake up. We're going to have a
          baby.

Grabbing his hand, she places it on her tummy...

                    SARAH (CONT'D)
          We're going to have a baby.

Ripping his hand away from her stomach...

                    HENRY
          You had to wake up a tired, hard
          working man just to say your
          pregnant?

Henry rolls over in bed, turning his back to Sarah.

Excitedly, She leaps from the bed.

13   KITCHEN

Sarah jolts down the hallway, through the living room, and to
the telephone in the kitchen.

Swiping the phone from the receiver, she dials a number and
waits impatiently.

A female voice answers.

                    SARAH
               (into phone)
          Anna...?

14   INT. ANNA'S LIVING ROOM- SAME TIME

                    ANNA
               This is she.

INTERCUT SARAH/ANNA

                    SARAH
                  (excited)
               Sarah here.

                    ANNA (V.O.)
               You better spill it, girl.

                    SARAH
               Well, you know I've been sick all
               week, right?

                    ANNA
               Yes. And...?

Sarah paces the floor.

                    SARAH
               And it's only been when I wake up
               in the morning.

                    ANNA (V.O.)
               Oh no you're--

                    SARAH
               Oh Yes I am.

          ANNA (V.O.)   SARAH (CONT'D)
     You're... Pregnant!   Pregnant!

                    ANNA
               Oh my goodness. Congratulations.

                    SARAH
               I know. Isn't this awesome.

Sarah freezes in her tracks, looking dumbfounded.

                    SARAH (CONT'D)
               Okay, okay... Now what?

                    ANNA
               What do you mean, "Now what?"

                    SARAH
               I mean, what do I do now?

>   ANNA (V.O.)
>   (sentimentally)
>   Sarah, now you get ready to enjoy
>   the greatest nine months of your
>   life.

15   INT. OBSTETRICIAN'S OFFICE- DAY

SARAH lays on an examination table waiting for her
obstetrician. ANNA sits in a bedside chair.

>   ANNA
>   Five months, and he hasn't made a
>   single doctor's visit with you?

Sarah is rubbing her belly.

>   SARAH
>   Oh you know Henry. He's either too
>   busy, or--

>   ANNA
>   Or too drunk.

Sarah becomes agitated.

>   SARAH
>   I don't want to talk about it right
>   now, Anna. If he doesn't want to be
>   a part of this, then just let him
>   be.

>   ANNA
>   Well if I was a man, I'd take a set
>   of wire cutters and--

>   DR. NICHOLAS
>   Mrs. Logan...

The obstetrician, DR. NICHOLAS (mid 40s), enters the room
with Sarah's patient chart. Closing the door behind him.

>   DR. NICHOLAS (CONT'D)
>   ...And how are we doing today?

>   ANNA
>   We're gettin' fat doc... how are
>   you?

Embarrassed, Sarah shoos her hand at Anna.

                    SARAH
          Oh, hush. He wasn't talking to you.
          I'm doing fine Dr. Nicholas.

The doctor briefly looks over the chart before laying it
down. He begins the examination. Pushing and feeling around
her stomach.

                    DR. NICHOLAS
          Have you been experiencing any
          discomfort lately?

Sarah quickly gives Anna the "Keep your mouth shut" look.

                    SARAH
          If you mean any *unusual*
          discomfort... no sir.

                    DR. NICHOLAS
          Wonderful.

The doctor slaps on the examination gloves, grabbing the gel
for the ultrasound.

Taking a seat on his stool next to the examination bed, he
applies the gel...

                    DR. NICHOLAS (CONT'D)
          This may feel a little cold.

Sarah becomes gitty.

                    SARAH
          Will we know today?

                    DR. NICHOLAS
              (smiling)
          Yes, Sarah. At five months we can
          identify the baby's gender.

Sarah reaches over, clutching Anna's hand.

The girlfriends stare intently at the monitor as the doctor
begins the ultrasound.

An intense moment of silence...

                    DR. NICHOLAS (CONT'D)
          Aha. Right there. Can you see it?

Sarah anxiously strains at the monitor before looking to Anna
for conformation. Anna's eyebrows raise as she gives a shrug.

The doctor points to a speck on the monitor.

18

                         DR. NICHOLAS (CONT'D)
                    Right there. Do you see that small
                    protrusion?

He looks back at Sarah with a smile.

                         DR. NICHOLAS (CONT'D)
                    That means you're going to have a
                    baby boy.

Sarah begins to weep. Anna springs to her feet, hugging
Sarah.

                         SARAH
                    It's a boy, Anna. A baby boy.

                         ANNA
                    I know. I saw his thingy.

Peeling off his latex gloves...

                         DR. NICHOLAS
                    Does this little boy have a name?

                         SARAH
                    Joshua. His name is Joshua.

                         DR. NICHOLAS
                    Well that's a great name for a baby
                    boy. Congratulations, Sarah. You
                    take care of yourself, and I'll see
                    you next visit.

The doctor turns to exit the room.

16   INT. LOGAN'S FAMILY KITCHEN- DAY

SARAH stands over the kitchen sink washing dishes. There is a
knock at the door.

With a look of concern, she rubs her almost-full-term tummy
while waddling to the front door. It's ANNA.

                         ANNA
                    Surprise!

Anna is standing on the front porch, holding as many
giftwrapped packages that a woman can possibly hold. Beside
her is an assembled baby swing and walker.

                         SARAH
                    Oh, Anna... you shouldn't have.

Sarah tries to give her a hug to no avail, due to the presents Anna is holding.

                    SARAH (CONT'D)
          Well, come on in.

Anna peaks over Sarah's shoulder into the house.

                    ANNA
          He still at work?

                    SARAH
          Or at the bar. Let me give you a
          hand with all this stuff.

17   INT. LOGAN'S FAMILY CABIN- LATER

In the living room, ANNA sits in a recliner and SARAH on the couch, surrounded by opened gift boxes and shredded wrapping paper.

Sarah holds (a Onesie) up in the air.

                    SARAH
          Anna, this is beautiful. How could
          you afford something like this?

                    ANNA
          It was easy. I made it. That's why
          all these clothes have little
          animal designs. I started making
          them before we knew the baby's
          gender.

                    SARAH
          But... how?

                    ANNA
              (facetiously)
          With something called a *sewing
          machine.*

                    SARAH
              (somberly)
          But I could never make something
          like this.

Anna approaches, pushing the empty gift boxes off the couch and onto the floor, sliding in next to Sarah.

                    ANNA
          Sarah, being a good mother is not
          about knowing how to sew.
              (MORE)

20

                    ANNA (CONT'D)
          Sewing is just something that some
          moms do, and some don't. (beat)
          Being a good mother is about...
          it's about knowing the perfect time
          to reach over in the middle of the
          night to gently rock the cradle.
          It's about knowing the difference
          between your babies' 'I'm hungry'
          cry, and his 'I don't feel good'
          cry. It's about coming home after a
          hard days work, just in time to
          start your second full-time job
          when you walk through the front
          door.

Sarah's lip begins to quiver as she blinks back the tears.

                    SARAH
          But what if I don't know how to do
          all that?

Anna takes Sarah by the hand.

                    ANNA
          Sarah, you're not Ethel. *You've*
          made all your doctor's visits.
          You've eaten healthy over the last
          eight months. You've done
          everything that a good mother is
          supposed to do. You'll do fine
          And I'll be right here with you
          every step of the way.

Sarah wipes a tear from her cheek.

                    SARAH
          I'm sorry. I've just been a little
          emotional. The baby hasn't been
          very active today, and it's gotten
          me worried.

                    ANNA
          Oh I'm sure everything's fine, you
          little worry wart. Just say your
          prayers when you go to bed tonight,
          and let the good Lord take care of
          the rest.

Anna tries to stand as Sarah clinches her hand.

                    SARAH
          Thank you Anna. Not just for the
          gifts, but for everything.

                    ANNA
          You know I wouldn't miss this for
          the world.

                    SARAH
          Will you call me tomorrow?

                    ANNA
          As soon as I get home from work.

Anna helps Sarah to her feet.

                    ANNA (CONT'D)
          But first, I'd better help you
          clean up this mess.

                    SARAH
          You've done enough already. Go home
          to your little boy, and I'll talk
          to you tomorrow.

                    ANNA
          Well you don't have to tell me
          twice.

Anna reaches down to grab her jacket.

                    ANNA (CONT'D)
          OH! I almost forgot. I always save
          the best for last.

Reaching into the jacket pocket, Anna pulls out a tiny,
giftwrapped box and hands it to Sarah.

Sarah peels back the wrapping paper, opens the box, and
retrieves a handcrafted wooden angel, bearing the name
JOSHUA.

                    ANNA (CONT'D)
          I know angels are your favorite.

                    SARAH
          And now I'll finally have one of my
          own.

Anna punches her in the shoulder.

                    SARAH (CONT'D)
          Ouch. What was that for?

                    ANNA
          For being sappy. I'll call you
          tomorrow.

Anna grabs her purse and rushes out the front door.

18   INT. LOGAN'S FAMILY CABIN- LATER

SARAH stands sideways, staring into the bathroom mirror at the reflection of the bump beneath her gown.

With a somewhat concerned look, she rubs her bump one last time before turning off the light and heading to bed alone.

19   BEDROOM

Crawling under the covers, SARAH places the handcrafted wooden angel onto the night stand, clicks off the lamp, lays back and stares up at the ceiling.

Patting her tummy...

                    SARAH
              My little angel.

She sighs, then CLOSES HER EYES.

20   INT. LOGAN'S FAMILY CABIN- LATER

SARAH OPENS HER EYES and frantically sits up in bed.

Henry lays next to her, passed out and snoring.

She shakes him.

                    SARAH
              Henry. Henry.

He doesn't budge.

She rolls out of bed, rushing to the telephone.

21   KITCHEN

SARAH grabs the phone and dials a number.

                    ANNA (V.O.)
                 (sleepy)
              Hello.

INTERCUT SARAH/ANNA

                         SARAH
                    (into phone)
               Anna, he's not moving!

                         ANNA (V.O.)
               Henry...?

                         SARAH
               No. The baby. He's not moving!

                         ANNA (V.O.)
               Okay. Sarah, I need you to try and
               calm down. Can you do that for me?

Sarah begins taking slow, deep breaths.

                         ANNA (V.O.)
               Good girl. When was the last time
               you can remember him moving?

Sarah closes her eyes tightly while frantically holding her
tummy.

                         SARAH
               Think. Think... two days. It's been
               two days.

                         ANNA (V.O.)
               Okay. Sarah, I know you've been
               eating very healthy, but now I want
               you to do something for me. This
               will give the baby lots of energy.

22   INT. LOGAN'S FAMILY CABIN- LATER

SARAH sits on the couch in her nightgown, gorging herself
with chocolate cake.

Beside her lay open boxes of MOONPIES and TWINKIES, with an
open can of RC Cola on the coffee table.

Finishing the piece of cake, she finger-swipes the leftover
icing off the plate, sucking it off like a Lolli-POP.

Reaching over, she grabs a Moonpie from its box. Peeling back
the rapper, she peers at it intently.

                         SARAH
               Yuck...

She chomps down as though she hasn't eaten in weeks.

24

There is a brief montage of Sarah pacing back and forth in her living room throughout the night. Constantly rubbing her tummy.

23   INT. LOGAN'S FAMILY CABIN- DAY

In the early morning hours, SARAH lies on the couch, staring down at her tummy. Praying.

                    SARAH
          God. I'll do anything. Just let my
          baby be okay.

Looking to the clock on the wall, she kicks her feet off the couch and quickly waddles to the kitchen telephone.

Dials a number.

                    SARAH (CONT'D)
               (into phone)
          Hello, this is Sarah... Sarah
          Logan.
               (listening)
          Well, I was wondering if I could
          come in to see Dr. Nicholas this
          morning?
               (listening)
          No, I don't have an appointment,
          but--
               (listening)
          Yes. Yes it's an emergency. My baby
          hasn't moved the past couple of
          days.
               (listening)

Sarah quickly glances back to the clock on the wall.

                    SARAH (CONT'D)
          Oh, absolutely. Yes... yes. I'll be
          right there.

Hanging up the phone, she rushes down the hallway.

24   BEDROOM

Grabbing her robe from the bedpost, she leans down to shake Henry. Pausing, she pulls her hand back, leaving him passed out in bed.

25   INT. OBSTETRICIAN'S OFFICE- DAY

SARAH is laying on the examination table as DR. NICHOLAS
applies the gel for the ultrasound.

                    DR. NICHOLAS
          So there hasn't been much movement
          as of late?

                    SARAH
          Not for a couple of days now.

                    DR. NICHOLAS
               (smiling)
          Well, there are definitely days
          when the baby is less active.

Sarah fearfully eyes the monitor as the ultrasound begins.

The doctor moves his hand slowly over her stomach. His hand
STOPS, then moves even slower. SLOWER.

His smile slowly evaporates. Hand stops.

                    SARAH
               (anxious)
          What's wrong?

                    DR. NICHOLAS
          Well, there doesn't seem to be a...

He begins to move the wand across her stomach again.

                    SARAH
          A what?

He stops. Heavy sigh.

                    DR. NICHOLAS
          A heartbeat. I'm so sorry, Sarah.
          Your baby is gone.

                    SARAH
          No! That can't happen!

Placing his hand back on her stomach, an image reappears on
the monitor.

Pointing to the monitor...

                    DR. NICHOLAS
               (sympathetically)
          There. That is the umbilical
          cord... wrapped around his neck.

                    SARAH
          No! No! No!

Sarah begins to wail.

                    DR. NICHOLAS
          I'm so sorry.
               (beat)
          Is there anyone you need me to
          contact?

She pauses long enough to shake her head, 'No'.

                    DR. NICHOLAS (CONT'D)
          Take all the time you need, Sarah.
          I'll go and make arrangements with
          the hospital across the street.

Sarah turns away from the doctor, opening her hand that has
been tightly clasped around a tiny, wooden angel, bearing the
name JOSHUA.

The angel slowly falls to the floor...

                    YOUNG ADULT FEMALE (V.O.)
          When she was a child, she would lie
          in her bed at night, praying for an
          angel to come and take her away;
          dreaming of what it must be like to
          soar through the heavens on a
          moonlit, starry night. Ironically,
          as a mother, that very dream had
          become her nightmare. For, the
          angel of whom she had so long
          awaited had seemingly just taken
          from her that which she loved most
          in this world- her baby boy.

26   INT. GENERAL HOSPITAL- SAME DAY

SARAH is crouched down in the corner of a hospital room,
clutching to her stomach through her patient gown. Wailing.

She is cornered by DOCTOR #2 (40-ISH) and several nurses.

                    SARAH
               (yelling)
          You're not taking my baby from me!

                    DOCTOR #2
          Sarah, just calm--

                    SARAH
          Don't tell me to calm down! This
          baby is all that's good in my life,
          and nobody has the right to take
          him from me.

The doctor motions to the nurses with his hand, signaling
'I've got this.' He slowly approaches and crouches before
her.

                    DOCTOR #2
          Sarah, I need you to listen to me
          very carefully.

She stubbornly turns her head away from his gaze.

                    DOCTOR #2 (CONT'D)
          Sarah. If you keep the baby any
          longer you could die.

She cups her hands over her ears.

                    SARAH
          No! No! No!

The doctor motions again for the nurses to stay back.

                    DOCTOR #2
          Sarah...

He leans forward, gently removing her hands from her ears.

                    DOCTOR #2 (CONT'D)
          Your baby has started to decompose
          inside your uterus. Please... He
          has to come out.

She finally makes eye contact with the doctor.

                    SARAH
              (whispering)
          Can I just keep him a while longer?

                    DOCTOR #2
          Of course you can. But only for a
          little while. Do you understand?

Sarah nods.

                    DOCTOR #2 (CONT'D)
          Okay. The nurses will help you back
          into bed, and I'll be back a little
          later.

27   INT. GENERAL HOSPITAL- NEXT DAY

SARAH, in a patient's gown, sitting in a wheelchair, stares
out her room window at nothing. Her eyes are emotionless.

In the b.g., we see the door to her room open. SARAH doesn't
flinch. The blurred image of a visitor enters.

The visitor approaches SARAH, leaning down and kissing her on
the head. It's ANNA.

                    ANNA (O.C.)
          Hey, Hun.

Unresponsive, Sarah continues to stare out the window as Anna
sits in a chair next to her.

                    ANNA (CONT'D)
          I stopped by the nursing home and
          spoke with your boss. She said to
          take all the time you need.

Sarah remains unresponsive.

                    ANNA (O.C.) (CONT'D)
          They're all praying for you, Sarah.
          We all are.

Sarah sighs in sarcasm, exhaling heavily through her
nostrils.

Still staring out the window...

                    SARAH
                (facetiously)
          Prayer...

Anna deflects the subtle sarcasm.

                    ANNA
          Yes, dear. We're all praying for
          you. Mrs. Phillips even--

                    SARAH
                (somberly)
          'Just say your prayers tonight when
          you go to bed, and let the *good*
          Lord take care of the rest.'

                    ANNA
          I... don't think I follow what
          you're--

> SARAH
> Isn't that what you said?

Sarah slowly turns her gaze toward Anna.

> SARAH (CONT'D)
> 'Just say your prayers and let the
> *good* Lord take care of the rest?'

Her lip quivers as she gazes back out the window.

> SARAH (CONT'D)
> *Good*... Anna? Is that what this is?
> The *goodness* of God?

Anna leans forward to take hold of Sarah's limp hand that hangs from the arm of the wheelchair.

> ANNA
> Now, Sarah...

Sarah jerks her hand away from Anna's grasp.

> SARAH
> No, Anna! Tell me! Is this the best
> He has to offer? Is this the
> goodness of God?

Sarah breaks. Her hands cradle her face, muffling her shrieks.

Anna remains speechless as tears streak down her cheeks.

> SARAH (CONT'D)
> (into hands)
> No... God... No! I promised you.

Sarah somewhat collects herself.

Staring again out the window...

> SARAH (CONT'D)
> You know, when I left the house to
> come see Dr. Nicholas, I prayed and
> I prayed. (beat) If I'm being
> punished for something I've done in
> the past...

Looking over to Anna...

> SARAH (CONT'D)
> Isn't Henry's beatings enough
> punishment?

Anna leaps toward her, cradling a sobbing Sarah as she melts into Anna's arms.

From outside the hospital window, we slowly ascend up and away, as if God had been peeking in on them.

> YOUNG ADULT FEMALE (V.O.)
> I've heard people say that, "Time can heal all wounds." But I've never heard them talk about the scars that are left behind, or the pain that is seemingly trapped just below the surface of the skin; like a disease, slowly eating away at the heart, until all that is left is a naked and battered soul.

28   EXT. CEMETERY- NEXT DAY

A Priest stands at one end of a tiny wooden box, reading from his Bible. There are ten chairs at the grave site. Eight are empty, with Anna and Ethel sitting in the other 2. Sarah stands over the tiny wooden box, holding a tiny, lifeless baby that is wrapped in a blanket.

With PUFFY, TEAR FILLED EYES, Sarah stares down into her arms, cradling her baby.

After one final kiss, she leans over, placing Joshua into the tiny, wooden box.

> YOUNG ADULT FEMALE (V.O.)
> There was a part of her that died that day. Every bone in her body wanted to follow baby Joshua into that grave.

After placing the baby into the wooden box, Sarah collapses to the ground. Anna races from her chair to comfort her. Ethel remains seated.

29   INT. THE LOGAN'S CABIN- NIGHT

SARAH sorts through stacks of clothes on the couch. Henry's clothes, she folds and places in a laundry basket. The baby's clothes, she folds and places in a box.

There is a knock at the front door.

SARAH approaches and cracks the door. It's ETHEL, now (60ish).

                    SARAH
          It's a little late don't you think?

                    ETHEL JACKSON
                    (smiling)
          Well, can't I visit my daughter?

Sarah curiously nods while opening the door.

30   INT. LOGAN FAMILY KITCHEN- LATER

With her back to Ethel, Sarah pours two cups of coffee. Ethel
sits at the kitchen table, smoking a cigarette, ending a
funny story...

                    ETHEL JACKSON
                    (laughing)
          ...Then your stepfather fell over
          the coffee table while he was
          chasing after the squirrel.

Sarah rolls her eyes while pouring the creamer.

Grabbing the cups, she joins Ethel at the table.

                    SARAH
          So what's up? You just come over to
          tell me about a dead squirrel?

Ethel's laughter fades as she points to Sarah, holding her
cigarette between her index and middle fingers.

                    ETHEL JACKSON
          You think Paul would ever commit
          suicide?

Sarah chokes on a sip of coffee...

                    SARAH
          Paul? Are you kidding?

                    ETHEL JACKSON
                    (chuckling)
          Oh, calm down. He just seems a
          little depressed lately. It's no
          big deal.

Sarah leans forward aggressively.

                    SARAH
          No big deal? This is Paul we're
          talking about. Your husband.

Ethel scowls at Sarah, taking a SLOW, EXTENDED DRAG from her
cigarette. Exhaling the smoke nonchalantly into Sarah's face.
Sarah shies back into her chair.

Ethel smirks.

                    ETHEL JACKSON
          Enough about Paul. How've you been?

                    SARAH
          Kind of excited, actually.

Sarah hops up and over to the kitchen sink, swiping an
ashtray from the window sill.

                    SARAH (CONT'D)
          I've started taking fertility
          pills.

Sarah sits back down, handing Ethel the ashtray.

                    ETHEL JACKSON
          No thanks. I've got one right here.

Ethel reaches her hand down into a box beside the table. She
pulls out a tiny, blue baby bottle, FLICKING the cigarette
ashes into it.

Sarah BITES DOWN on the corner of her lip. Hiding her fury.

                    ETHEL JACKSON (CONT'D)
          Do you think Henry wants to go
          through this again?

Sarah freezes, like a five-year old being scorned.

Ethel points her two-fingered, cigarette jab at Sarah again.

                    ETHEL JACKSON (CONT'D)
          Look at you. It's been four months,
          and you're still sulking.

She flicks another ash into the baby bottle.

Sarah's jaws clinch as the tears well in her eyes.

                    SARAH
          Mother... but I've been praying--

                    ETHEL JACKSON
          Praying? Do you think God's
          listening to you- a little girl who
          ran off to marry that poor excuse
          of a man who, as we speak is passed-
          out in your bed.

Ethel drops the butt of her cigarette into the baby bottle.

Sarah clears the table with one swipe of her arm. Coffee cups
EXPLODE against the wall as she springs to her feet, pointing
to the front door...

                    SARAH
          Get out, Ethel!

Ethel just sits there, smirking.

                    SARAH (CONT'D)
          I said get out.

Ethel grabs her purse, slowly backing towards the door.

                    ETHEL JACKSON
          The baby's dead, Sarah.

Sarah swipes a glass from the kitchen strainer, hurling it at
Ethel as she exits, shattering against the door.

31   INT. LOGAN'S FAMILY KITCHEN- DAY

The next morning, dressed in scrubs, SARAH places a plate of
breakfast before HENRY, then sits across from him at the
kitchen table, sipping on a cup of coffee, watching as he is
smacks it down- bite after bite.

                    HENRY
          What was all that racket about last
          night?

                    SARAH
          Oh, mother stopped by.

                    HENRY
          Ethel? That's a first.

                    SARAH
          She's just worried about Paul.

With a mouthful of food...

                    HENRY
               (chuckles)
          He finally wise up and leave her?

                    SARAH
          It's not funny, Henry. She's
          worried about him committing
          suicide.

                    HENRY
          Can ya blame him? I'm surprised
          he's made it this long.

                    SARAH
          I guess you make a good point. It's
          just that... I don't know, it just
          seemed like she really didn't care;
          like she had no compassion for him.

Henry briefly pauses from his feeding frenzy...

                    HENRY
          And that surprises you?

                    SARAH
          I don't know.

Sarah moves to the kitchen sink, dumping the remainder of her
coffee, rinsing the cup.

                    SARAH (CONT'D)
          It's just that she's never been by
          to visit. Something just didn't
          seem right.

Henry grabs his plate, walking over to the sink.

                    HENRY
          Kinda like how these eggs don't
          seem right. You ever gonna learn
          how to cook?

He drops the plate into the sink.

                    HENRY (CONT'D)
          If you'd spend more time worrying
          about what *you're* supposed to be
          doing, and less time worrying about
          what Ethel's doing, then maybe
          you'd be able to cook your husband
          a decent meal.

                    SARAH
          I've got to get to work.

The phone rings.

> HENRY
> You call that work... playin' games
> with old folks and wiping their
> snotty noses?

Sarah answers the phone.

> SARAH
> (into phone)
> Hello.

> HENRY (CONT'D)
> When are you gonna become a
> real nurse...

> SARAH
> (into phone)
> Yes, this Sarah.
> (listening)

> HENRY (CONT'D)
> ...And start making real
> money?

She places her hand over the receiver.

> SARAH
> (to Henry)
> I can't hear.

Henry shoos his hand while exiting the kitchen...

> HENRY
> And ya can't cook.

> SARAH
> (into phone)
> I'm sorry. Yes, this is Sarah
> Logan.
> (listening)

Sarah's countenance becomes that of shock.

> SARAH (CONT'D)
> Oh my God. Is he already there at
> the hospital?
> (listening)
> Okay. Yes, I'll be right there.

Sarah grabs her purse and storms out the front door.

32   INT. GENERAL HOSPITAL- DAY

SARAH rushes through the sliding glass doors of the ER. Two
police officers, CAPTAIN BERNARD (mid 50s) and LIEUTENANT
CAPSHAW (mid 30s) are standing with ETHEL at the nurses
station, questioning her.

SARAH and ETHEL share a quick glance.

ANNA jumps from her seat and rushes to meet SARAH.

                    SARAH
          Anna?

                    ANNA
          I happened to be driving by when
          they were loading him into the
          ambulance. So I followed them here
          and had them call you as soon as we
          arrived.

                    SARAH
          What happened? What's going on?

Anna takes Sarah by the arm, leading her to take a seat in
the waiting area.

                    ANNA
               (quietly)
          From what I can gather, Ethel found
          Paul lying in the back yard this
          morning, apparently having shot
          himself with a handgun.

Sarah glances across the room, again making eye contact with
Ethel, who is still being questioned by the officers.

                    ANNA (CONT'D)
          Why do you not seem surprised?

                    SARAH
          So how is he?

                    ANNA
          He's lost a lot of blood, Sarah,
          after apparently laying in the back
          yard most of the night. He's in
          surgery right now, but they said he
          has serious stomach injuries--

                    SARAH
          Stomach? Why would you shoot
          yourself in the stomach if you were
          trying to commit suicide?

The two officers approach Sarah.

                    CAPTAIN BERNARD
          Mrs. Logan... Sarah, is it?

> SARAH
> Yes. I'm Sarah Logan.

Captain Bernard is holding a pencil and a pocket booklet.

> CAPTAIN BERNARD
> I'm Captain Bernard, and this is
> Lieutenant Capshaw.

> LIEUTENANT CAPSHAW
> Ma'am.

> CAPTAIN BERNARD
> We were just needing to ask you a
> few questions if that's alright?

> SARAH
> Sure. Anything.

> CAPTAIN BERNARD
> Now, your mother, Ethel, says that
> she was with you last night. Can
> you corroborate her statement?

> SARAH
> Well, she did stop by last night
> for--

> ETHEL JACKSON (O.C.)
>   (shouting)
> I said no!

Ethel shoves a doctor, and jabs her finger at a priest.

> ETHEL JACKSON (CONT'D)
> No one gets in to see my husband.
> Not even you, Father Jacobs.

She casts an evil glare across the room at Sarah.

> ETHEL JACKSON (CONT'D)
> No one!

Ethel turns, disappearing down the ER hallway.

33   EXT. GENERAL HOSPITAL- NIGHT

Sarah and Anna sit outside the ER entrance. Sarah, still in
scrubs, is lighting up a cigarette.

A YOUNG NURSE rushes out the glass sliding doors of the ER.

                    YOUNG NURSE
          Excuse me. Sarah, you're needed
          inside.

Sarah flicks her cigarette into the night air.

34   INT. GENERAL HOSPITAL- SAME NIGHT

SARAH and ANNA chase after the nurse, down the hallway and to
the doorway of Paul's ICU room, where an OLD DOCTOR (60s) and
a priest, FATHER JACOBS (60s) are waiting.

                    SARAH
          What's going on?

                    OLD DOCTOR
          I'm sorry, Sarah. Paul didn't make
          it. Of course you know Father
          Jacobs... and please give your
          mother my regards.

The doctor gives Sarah a comforting pat on the shoulder while
walking away.

                    FATHER JACOBS
          I'm truly sorry to be meeting under
          these conditions, Sarah.

                    SARAH
          Is she still in there?

                    FATHER JACOBS
          And she still won't allow anyone to
          come in. I was thinking we might
          just pray together out here in the
          hallway?

                    ANNA
          Absolutely.

Sarah begins to slowly back-peddle.

                    SARAH
          Actually, I'd better be getting
          home.

                    ANNA
          Sarah...?

                    SARAH
          Anna, Just let me go.

Sarah rushes away, leaving the priest and Anna.

> ANNA
> (loudly)
> You can't keep running, Sarah.

35   INT. GERIATRICS CENTER- DAY

SARAH, dressed in scrubs, cries out as she rushes into MRS. PHILLIPS' room to help her up from the floor.

> SARAH
> Mrs. Phillips! Are you okay?

> MRS. PHILLIPS
> Oh Hun, you're my angel sent from
> heaven.

Sarah takes Mrs. Phillips by the hand and arm, helping her to balance while she stands...

> SARAH
> (smiling)
> Well, no one has ever referred to
> me as an angel before.

She helps Mrs. Phillips back into bed, tucking her in snuggly.

> MRS. PHILLIPS
> Well, an angel is one of those
> ministering spirits whom has been
> sent to serve those who will
> inherit salvation.

> SARAH
> Pssh. Doesn't look like I'll be
> going to heaven.

> MRS. PHILLIPS
> Oh, child. Why would you say such a
> thing?

Sarah hastily avoids eye contact...

> SARAH
> Because God has never sent me an
> angel.

Mrs. Phillips senses her hostility and changes the subject.

> MRS. PHILLIPS
> I nearly forgot. That friend of
> yours... the electrician gal?

                    SARAH
          Anna?

                    MRS. PHILLIPS
          She was in here last evening
          lookin' for ya. Seemed disappointed
          you'd already gone for the day.

Sarah's countenance is one of shame as she draws the window
curtains together.

                    SARAH
          Yeah, I haven't seen or spoken to
          her in about a month... since,
          well, my step-dad.

                    MRS. PHILLIPS
          They ever find out what really
          happened?

                    SARAH
          The Sheriff said it was a suicide,
          and left it at that.

                    MRS. PHILLIPS
          And what about your friend?

Sarah finishes drawing the curtains, turning back to Mrs.
Phillips...

                    SARAH
          Anna? What do you mean?

                    MRS. PHILLIPS
          Have you told her the good news?

Sarah appears confused...

                    SARAH
          What good news?

                    MRS. PHILLIPS
          That you're with child again.

                    SARAH
          BUT...! How...?

With a smile of joy, Sarah rushes back to Mrs. Phillips.

> MRS. PHILLIPS
> (chuckling)
> I spect there had to be a reason
> you been sick in my bathroom bout
> every other morning. I'd also spect
> your friend would like to know.

> SARAH
> Well I'd *spect* you're probably
> right.

Sarah makes her way to leave the room.

> MRS. PHILLIPS
> And Sarah, don't give up child. For
> some have entertained angels never
> knowing it.

36   INT. COFFEE SHOP- DAY

The beginning of a montage.

Sarah and Anna sit across a small table from one another.

Anna leaps from her chair and swallows Sarah up with a hug,
while Sarah, laughing, is trying to stop her from making such
a big scene in the coffee shop.

37   INT. GENERAL HOSPITAL- DAY

Sarah lays on a gurney in the delivery room, pushing with all
her might.

Anna stands alongside Sarah, holding her hand, with painful
facial expressions caused by Sarah's tight grip.

> YOUNG ADULT FEMALE (V.O.)
> On December 12th, 1983, Sarah gave
> birth to a healthy baby boy. Noah
> Logan came into this world weighing
> 7 pounds and 14 ounces, and was 20
> inches long.

38   INT. GENERAL HOSPITAL- SAME DAY

Sarah lays in the hospital bed holding her newborn baby,
while Anna is taking pictures.

                    YOUNG ADULT FEMALE (V.O.)
          Though Henry managed to finally
          arrive at the hospital, he had made
          it clear that he didn't want to be
          in the delivery room... which was
          fine. He actually never held Noah
          in his arms until he was taken home
          a few days later.

39   INT. LOGAN'S FAMILY HOME- NIGHT

        Sarah walks through the front door of her house in her work
        scrubs, carrying baby Noah in one arm, along with a diaper
        bag draped over her shoulder and a bag of groceries in the
        other arm.

        Kicking the door closed with her foot, her shoulders slouch
        with exhaustion when she sees what a mess the house is in.

                    YOUNG ADULT FEMALE (V.O.)
          She was finally busy being a
          mother. Everything had become
          different. And though her work load
          had doubled, she could have cared
          less.

40   INT. LOGAN'S FAMILY KITCHEN- DAY

        Sarah stands at the kitchen sink washing dishes and baby
        bottles, while at the same time trying to quieten a screaming
        baby Noah, who lays in a baby seat atop the kitchen counter
        by the sink.

                    YOUNG ADULT FEMALE (V.O.)
          Extra dishes. Extra laundry. Lack
          of sleep. She loved it. The only
          thing that could have made her life
          more difficult was...

41   INT. LOGAN'S FAMILY HOME- NIGHT

        Sarah walks through the front door of her house in her work
        scrubs, carrying a one-year old baby Noah, a diaper bag and a
        bag of groceries.

        Kicking the door closed with her foot, her shoulders slouch
        with exhaustion when she sees what a mess the house is in.
        Sporting another baby-bump.

                    YOUNG ADULT FEMALE (V.O.)
          ...Another baby.

42   INT. GENERAL HOSPITAL- DAY

An exhausted Sarah lays in a hospital bed, holding her
newborn son. Anna is snapping photos.

                    YOUNG ADULT FEMALE (V.O.)
              On April 6th, 1985, she gave birth
              to another healthy baby boy. Eli
              Logan came into this world weighing
              7 pounds, 6 and a half ounces, and
              was 21 inches long. And oh how
              those boys grew so quickly
              together.

43   INT. LOGAN'S FAMILY HOME- DAY

Sarah sits in a rocker, with baby Eli asleep in one arm and
eighteen-month old Noah asleep in the other.

44   EXT. LOGAN'S FAMILY HOME- DAY

A three-year old Noah and two-year old Eli play in a
toddler's swimming pool in the front yard. Sarah sits,
laughing, watching from a chair on the front porch.

45   EXT. FOXWOODS UNIVERSITY- NIGHT

We see a campus building, reading FOXWOODS UNIVERSITY.

46   INT. FOXWOODS UNIVERSITY- NIGHT

Sarah sits in a room filled with men and women who are
wearing scrubs. She takes notes as the professor lectures.

47   INT. LOGAN'S FAMILY HOME- NIGHT

Sarah enters through the front door, wearing scrubs, with a
backpack over her shoulder and carrying a bag of groceries.

The two boys run to her, grabbing each of her legs. Sarah's
laughter quickly fades as she sees Henry passed out on the
couch, and an empty whiskey bottle lying on the floor next to
him.

48   INT. LOGAN'S FAMILY HOME- EARLY MORNING

Sarah, in a bathrobe, excitedly sits in the living room floor
beside a Christmas tree, alongside a four-year-old Noah and
three-year-old Eli who are joyously tearing into their
Christmas presents.

Amid the excitement, she jumps up and rushes to her bedroom
door, peeking in on a passed out Henry. With a look of
disappointment, she quietly closes the door and goes back to
the Christmas fun.

49   EXT. SPENCER'S CAR GARAGE (1989)

Anna's husband, SPENCER (30ish), is under the hood of a
vintage car. ANNA and her son, DONOVAN (5), sit off to the
side on fold-out chairs.

SARAH, ELI and Noah drive up to the front of the garage and
park. Hopping out of the car, they approach SPENCER.

Holding open the carburetor with a screwdriver, SPENCER yells
to MATTHEW (30ish) and handsome, sitting behind the wheel...

                    SPENCER
          Try it again Matt.

The engine cranks but doesn't turn over.

                    SARAH
          You still trying to get this old
          thing started, Spence?

Spencer chuckles...

                    SPENCER
          This *old thing*, is a 1962 Impala
          SS. And yes.

Anna hops up from her chair, kissing Spencer on the cheek...

                    ANNA
          Yep. He promised he'd have it
          running by our anniversary.

                    ELI
          Mommy, can we go play with Donovan?

                    SARAH
          You bet.

The three boys rush off into mischief.

                    SARAH (CONT'D)
          But stay close, we won't be here
          long.

                    ANNA
                (jokingly)
          Yeah. Heaven forbid your mother
          have a life away from home.

Sarah punches Anna in the shoulder...

                    SARAH
          Oh, whatever.

                    ANNA
          Just sayin', I know a huge Italian
          man who can take care of the
          problem.

                    SARAH
          Well, right now I'm just looking
          for a man to take care of my oil
          leak.

Matthew hops out of the car...

                    MATTHEW
          I can help.

Anna becomes gitty...

                    ANNA
          Of course he can. Come around here,
          Matt.

Sarah blushes.

                    SARAH
          Anna...

                    ANNA
                (to Matthew)
          This is my best friend, Sarah.
                (to Sarah)
          Sarah, this is Spencer's friend,
          Matthew.

Definitely a connection between the two as their eyes meet.

Matthew gets tongue-tide...

                    MATTHEW
          I'm... uh...

                    ANNA
          ...Uh doctor, who likes to restore
          vintage cars in his free time.

As he reaches for a handshake, Sarah snaps out of her trance-
like state, becoming almost rigid...

                    SARAH
          Well, I don't care who does it, I
          just can't be--

Anna breaks in with her best "Henry" imitation...

47
                    ANNA
          Leakin' oil all over Henry's
          driveway.

                    SARAH

          Anna--

                    ANNA
          No need to thank me.

                    SARAH
          I was going to say, 'You're such a
          dork.'

                    SPENCER
          Absolutely.

Spencer purposely spins a play-on-words.

                    ANNA
             (to Spencer)
          You're agreeing with her?

He retracts as though it was an accident.

                    SPENCER
          No, babe. I was just telling Sarah,
          'Absolutely. Just drop it with me
          one day next week, and either me or
          Matt will getcha fixed up.'

50   EXT. LOGAN'S FAMILY HOME- SAME DAY

SARAH, ELI and Noah exit the car.

                    SARAH
          Hey, you two go put on your swim-
          trunks while I get the groceries.

                         ELI
          Are you going to fill the pool,
          Mommy?

                         SARAH
          You bet.

The boys race to the house as Sarah opens the trunk of the
car.

While retrieving the brown paper bags of groceries, one of
the bags rip. Fruit rolls everywhere.

                         SARAH (CONT'D)
          You've got to be kidding.

She begins picking up the spilled apples and oranges.

Suddenly, she hears a scream coming from one of her boys in
the house. She drops everything.

51   INT. LOGAN'S FAMILY HOME- SAME TIME

Noah is on the couch crying, while ELI sits beside him in
fear. With beer in hand and slurred speech, HENRY lashes
out...

                         HENRY
          This is what happens when you don't
          mind me, boys.

Sarah busts through the front door.

                         SARAH
          What's going on?

She rushes over to Noah.

                         HENRY
             (to Sarah)
          I'm not gonna tell him again to
          pick up his toys... and where've
          you been all day?

Sarah frantically searches Noah, feeling for fractures in his
arms and shoulders, finally spotting his rosey-red cheek.

She pulls Noah and Eli in close.

                         SARAH
             (muttering)
          He's just a little boy.

                    HENRY
          What did you say?

Henry staggers toward Sarah, flinging his half-empty beer can
across the room...

                    HENRY (CONT'D)
          What did you say to me?

Grabbing her by the shoulders, he stands Sarah up.

                    SARAH
               (fearlessly)
          I said, "He's just a child!"

Henry hurls her into a wall, before stumbling to the floor
himself.

                    HENRY
          Don't you sass me, woman.

Sarah jumps to her feet, grabs up both Eli and Noah and
rushes to the bedroom, locking the door behind her.

Henry follows. Palm-slapping the door...

                    HENRY (CONT'D)
          If you've got somethin' to say to
          me, then come out here and say it
          to my face.

52   BEDROOM

Sarah lays on the bed, tightly clinging to her sons.

Henry bangs again...

                    HENRY (O.S.)
          Sarah! Sarah! Maybe it's best you
          just stay in there the rest of the
          day... I'm goin' out.

Eli raises and cuddles Sarah's face in his hands...

                    ELI
          Don't cry mommy.

She pulls Eli close and rests her chin atop his head.

Through angry tears...

                    SARAH
          Oh my love, everything's going to
          be just fine.

She kisses Noah atop his head, glancing again at his cheek...

                    SARAH (CONT'D)
          Are you okay, honey? Are you okay?

Noah gives a tearful nod of reassurance.

                    SARAH (CONT'D)
          Mommy will never let that happen to
          you again.

Eli raises back up...

                    ELI
          Mommy, who's Jesus?

Sarah pulls he and Noah tightly back into her bosom, as she
hastily looks to the ceiling...

                    SARAH
          He's no one, honey. Mommy's going
          to protect you from now on... both
          of you.

Noah reaches over, taking Eli by the hand.

53   EXT. LOGAN FAMILY HOME- LATER

It's late. Midnight dark. SARAH quietly closes the front door
behind her. NOAH, in pajamas, carries his blanky. SARAH takes
him by the hand. Eli, also in PJ's, asleep on Sarah's
shoulder.

SARAH is met in the front yard by ANNA and VINCE (30s), a
huge Italian man.

SARAH, shocked to see the man, gives ANNA a look...

                    SARAH
               (quietly)
          Really, Anna?

                    ANNA
          You know I don't play around. This
          is Vince.

With his Italian accent...

                    VINCE
          You got nothin' to worry about,
          Sarah.

                    SARAH
          No kidding. He's passed out, as
          usual.

                    ANNA
          Vince, watch the front door.

                    VINCE
          You got it.

Leaving Vince behind, they scurry toward Sarah's car...

                    ANNA
          So everything's set with the
          apartment?

                    SARAH
          We should be good--

                    ANNA
          And you and the boys have plenty of
          clothes?

                    SARAH
          I've packed plent--

                    ANNA
          What about food? And toys? And
          Money?

Sarah stops in her tracks.

                    SARAH
          Anna. We're going to be fine.

                    ANNA
          I know, I know. I'm sorry. I
          just...

                    SARAH
          Me too, Anna. Me too.

Anna reaches into her back pocket and pulls out a white
envelope.

                    ANNA
          Look, it's not much, but it's
          something.

                    SARAH
          Anna, I can't--

                    ANNA
          Shut it, woman. This is what family
          does.

Anna slides the envelope into Sarah's purse.

                    SARAH
          I'll call you when I get to
          Durango.

                    ANNA
          Yeah, you'd better. Now get outta
          here while I go get the Italian
          watchdog off your lawn.

Anna turns to walk away.

                    SARAH
          Hey, Anna...

Anna looks back.

                    SARAH (CONT'D)
          ...That's not my lawn.

54   INT. SARAH'S APARTMENT- NIGHT

     SUPERIMPOSE
                    DURANGO, CO, 6 MONTHS
                    LATER

     In her humble apartment, with the cordless telephone to her
     ear, SARAH sits at a tiny kitchen table with Noah and Eli,
     piecing together a jigsaw puzzle amidst their just-finished
     dinner plates.

                    SARAH
               (into phone)
          Yes, Anna. Didn't we have this
          conversation yesterday?
               (listening)
          Exactly. Then I told you the boys
          and I had a wonderful Thanksgiving
          dinner and--
               (listening)
          Would you please stop worrying?
          We're doing fine. We're all excited
          about starting this new chapter in
          our lives.
               (listening)

Sarah stacks the dirty dinner plates and heads toward the kitchen sink.

                    SARAH (CONT'D)
         (softly)
    Not that it's any of your business,
    but, yes. Matthew and I have been
    out a couple of times.
         (listening)
    I know. He's such a gentleman.

Sarah drops the dishes in the sink before swooping over to swipe the chocolate ice cream from the freezer.

                    SARAH (CONT'D)

    Are you crazy? I'm not looking to jump
    into anything serious right now. I
    just need some adult interaction to
    help... keep my sanity.
         (listening)

As though it's routine, she pulls two bowls down from the cabinet and the ice cream scoop from the strainer, before briefly pausing with a look of disgust...

                    SARAH (CONT'D)
    Do we *really* have to talk about
    him?

She begins scooping the ice cream into the bowls.

                    SARAH (CONT'D)
    Of course. He's still the same ole
    Henry- Calling at all hours of the
    night, with no regard to the boys
    being asleep... dropping in
    unexpectedly; drunk of course...
    and seemingly becoming best friends
    with Ethel.
         (listening)

She pulls two spoons from a drawer, traps the phone between her shoulder and ear, and delivers the nightly treat to Noah and Eli.

                    SARAH (CONT'D)
         (to the boys)
    Mommy has your favorite.

She places the bowls on the table.

          NOAH   ELI
Ice cream!   Ice cream!

                    SARAH
               (into phone)
          No. He hasn't lifted a hand to help
          with Eli's medical bills.
               (listening)

Sarah kisses Noah atop his head, then Eli, as they dig in.

Sarah remains focused on Eli.

                    SARAH (CONT'D)
               (into phone)
          Poor, little guy. He's been
          battling sinusitis and
          mononucleosis all fall, and now the
          doctor is saying he needs tubes in
          his ears.

Sarah feels something on the back, right side of Eli's neck,
bending down for a closer look.

                    SARAH (CONT'D)
               (into phone)
          Hey, I'll have to call you back in
          a bit.
               (listening)
          You too.

Sarah hits the off button, lays the phone on the table.

                    SARAH (CONT'D)
          Eli, honey, what's this bump on the
          back of your neck? Did you run into
          something?

Between slurps of ice cream...

                    ELI
          Nope.

                    SARAH
          Does it hurt when mommy touches it?

                    ELI
          Nope.

                    SARAH
          What about now?

                    ELI
          Uh-huh.

                    SARAH
          Well, does it hurt when I do...
          this?

Sarah tickles him in the ribs as he cackles out...

                    ELI
          No... Mommy.

55   INT. DURANGO MALL- DAY

It's Christmas time. SARAH, ELI and NOAH sit at a table in
the food court. The boys joyously lapping up their ice cream
cones while SARAH sips on her milkshake.

The studious Noah inquires...

                    NOAH
          Mommy, do you believe in Santa?

Sarah's eyes bulge as she gulps the milkshake.

                    SARAH
          Well of course, honey. Why would
          you ask me that?

                    NOAH
          We were reading a book at school
          about how the mean Grinch stole
          Christmas, and Billy Dougan said
          that Santa wasn't real.

                    SARAH
          Not real? Then where do all the
          Christmas presents come from?

                    NOAH
          He says they come from Martians in
          outer space.

                    SARAH
               (to self)
          Well that's more believable.
               (to Noah)
          Well Billy Dougan doesn't know what
          he's talking about.

                    NOAH
          Don't worry, Mom. That's what I
          told him. (beat) Mommy, do you
          believe in angels?

Hiding behind another sip of milkshake, Sarah retains a
serious countenance before letting out a fake giggle...

                    SARAH
          Where are all these questions
          coming from, you little turkey?
          Where do you hear about this stuff?

Innocently licking his cone...

                    NOAH
          Last night Eli woke me up and asked
          if I believed in angels.

Sarah curiously glances at Eli.

                    NOAH (CONT'D)
          Well, do ya...?

Biting down on her lip, masking her bitterness, Sarah lets
out another giggle...

                    SARAH
          I'll tell you what I believe. I
          believe your ice cream is gonna
          melt if you two don't get to
          lickin.

                    ELI
          Mommy, I don't feel so good.

She places the back of her hand on Eli's forehead...

                    SARAH
          Oh, honey, you're starting to run
          fever again. How bout we go home
          and mommy will bake some
          gingerbread cookies?

Noah slides out of his seat, placing his arm around Eli...

                    NOAH
               (nurturing)
          And we can even watch *your* favorite
          cartoons, Eli.

56   INT. SARAH'S APARTMENT- NIGHT

         SUPERIMPOSE
                    January, 1990

SARAH sneaks into the front door of her dimly lit apartment, wearing scrubs, a backpack over one shoulder, a purse, and carrying a single brown paper bag of groceries.

She finds HANNAH, the baby sitter, (20ish), with an appearance as though she is mature for her age, lying on the couch watching a silent television while reading a book.

The boys cuddled together, asleep, on a pallet in the floor.

SARAH places the groceries on the kitchen table. HANNAH hops up to greet her.

                    SARAH
               (quietly)
          I am so sorry, Hannah. The
          professor's lecture ran way over.

Hannah shoos her hand at Sarah...

                    HANNAH
          You know that's never a problem,
          Sarah.

                    SARAH
          I'd give anything to be able to
          afford one of those new... car
          phone thingies.

Sarah pulls a folded up twenty out of her purse...

                    SARAH (CONT'D)
          You're worth so much more to me
          than what I can afford... were they
          good?

They look to the sleeping children.

                    HANNAH
          As always.

                    SARAH
          And Eli?

Hannah grimaces...

                    HANNAH
          His temp stayed right at 100
          degrees all evening. Poor little
          guy.

                    SARAH
          Yeah. Almost seven months, and they
          still can't figure it out.

Hannah grabs her purse off the coat stand by the front door, while Sarah quietly twists the knob to open it.

> HANNAH
> Lord willing, they'll figure it out
> soon enough.

> SARAH
> (facetiously)
> Huh, like He really cares.

Hannah is stunned at the remark. Sarah quickly changes the tone, giving a hug...

> SARAH (CONT'D)
> Thank you again for all your help.

> HANNAH
> Anytime.

57   EXT. FRONT DOOR

> SARAH
> Oh, and by the way, over the last
> couple of months- when watching the
> boys... do you read to them?

> HANNAH
> Oh, yeah. They love Dr. Seuss.

> SARAH
> But have you ever read, like... the
> Bible or anything like that to
> them... anything about angels?

Hannah ponders...

> HANNAH
> No. Not that I can recall.

> SARAH
> Just wondering. Thanks again, and
> have a good night.

58   INT. FRONT DOOR

Sarah eases the door shut, turns the lock, leans back and reflects.

59   INT. DURANGO HOSPITAL ER- DAY (FEBRUARY)

SARAH comes flying through the sliding glass doors carrying
Eli, as Noah follows close behind.

Approaching the OLD NURSE at the help desk...

                    OLD NURSE
          May I help you?

                    SARAH
          Yes. It's my son. His fever spiked
          overnight, and I haven't been able
          to get it back down.

                    OLD NURSE
          And who's his pediatrician?

                    SARAH
          Dr. Owens.

The nurse hands Sarah a clipboard.

                    OLD NURSE
          Fill this out, dear, and I'll let
          him know you're here.

60   INT. DURANGO HOSPITAL- LATER

In an examination room, SARAH sits in a chair cuddling a sick
Eli. NOAH is standing across the room, staring at a picture
on the wall.

                    NOAH
          Mommy, what's that?

                    SARAH
          That's an ear, sweetie.

                    NOAH
          It doesn't look like an ear.

                    SARAH
          No, honey. That's the *inside* of an
          ear.

                    NOAH
          Is that what the doctor sees with
          his flashlight?

                    DR. OWENS
          That's exactly what we see, young
          man.

DR. OWENS (50ish), and short, enters, accompanied by DR. JAMES (50ish) and tall. Each wearing a lab coat.

Intimidated, Noah rushes over to Sarah's side.

> DR. OWENS (CONT'D)
> A little shy, are we?

Dr. James hands Dr. Owens a clipboard.

> DR. OWENS (CONT'D)
> Mrs. Logan, this is Dr. James, one
> of my colleagues.

Dr. James and Sarah give one another a nod.

Dr. Owens rolls a stool towards Sarah and sits down in front of her. As he looks through Eli's charts, Sarah notices Dr. James waiting by the door, seemingly annoyed.

> DR. OWENS (CONT'D)
> I'm going to prescribe him a
> different antibiotic this time. It
> appears he's having another bout
> with sinusitis--

> SARAH
> Sinusitis! That's your diagnosis...
> again?

> DR. OWENS
> Now, Mrs. Logan--

> SARAH
> No, Dr. Owens.

Sarah lowers her voice, realizing she's still holding Eli.

> SARAH (CONT'D)
> It's been seven months. We've seen
> three different doctors, a
> pediatrician, an ear, nose and
> throat specialist, and two general
> practitioners. He's had tubes
> placed in his ears, and you've had
> him on several different
> antibiotics, and now your
> prescribing yet another?
> Something's not right.

> DR. JAMES
> I agree Mrs. Logan...

Dr. James approaches...

60

>   DR. JAMES (CONT'D)
>   ...Which is why I requested to
>   accompany Dr. Owens today.

The two doctors begin to bicker.

>   DR. OWENS
>   Mrs. Logan, Dr. James has no
>   grounds or evidence to backup--

>   DR. JAMES
>   No evidence? The child has been
>   sick for nearly seven months--

>   DR. OWENS
>   Then what would you suggest,
>   *doctor*?

>   DR. JAMES
>   How about trying something
>   different... retracing our steps...
>   looking back on previous tests to
>   see if there's something we've
>   missed.

>   SARAH
>   Gentlemen.

Sarah springs from the chair, taking Noah by the hand.

>   SARAH (CONT'D)
>   You will not argue in front of my
>   children.

Leaning forward, eye to eye with Dr. Owens...

>   SARAH (CONT'D)
>   I don't care how you do it, just
>   figure it out.

61   INT. SARAH'S APARTMENT- SAME DAY

It's late. SARAH and NOAH walk through the front. Eli lay
asleep on Sarah's shoulder.

The phone is RINGING off the wall.

>   SARAH
>   Noah, could you please close the
>   door behind us.

Sarah gently lays Eli down on the couch. Noah crouches down
and rests his head upon Eli's.

                    NOAH
         Is he going to be okay, mommy?

The phone is still RINGING.

                    SARAH
         Absolutely, my love.

Kisses Noah on the head...

                    SARAH (CONT'D)
         Can you take care of brother while
         mommy answers the phone?

                    NOAH
         Ab..so..lutely.

Sarah jolts toward the annoying, repetitive ringing.

                    SARAH
              (into phone)
         Hello...

She hears only a busy signal. Hangs up the phone, and
sluggishly strolls back and settles on the floor next to
Noah, stroking his hair.

Noah quietly watches as his baby brother sleeps.

                    SARAH (CONT'D)
         What a day. (beat) You are such a
         trooper, son... and so much more
         brave than any other little boy I
         know. Your the best big brother in
         the whole world.

Noah continues to sit quietly, clutching onto Eli's hand.

                    SARAH (CONT'D)
         Mommy's going to take a quick
         shower, then I'll make us some
         dinner.

62   BATHROOM

Sarah removes her rings and wristwatch, placing them on the
sink. When removing her necklace, she suddenly catches a
glimpse of the woman in the mirror.

Leaning into the reflection, she examines her bloodshot eyes
that rest atop the puffy, dark bags that rest beneath.

Above her reflection, she spots the blurred image of a picture hanging on the wall behind her. Spinning around, she slowly removes the picture from the wall. It's Noah and Eli.

Clutching it tightly to her chest, she turns, slides down the wall. Sobbing.

63   INT. SARAH'S APARTMENT- DAY

BLACK SCREEN.

                    ANNA (O.S.)
          Oh... my... sweet Lord and Savior.

Looking up through blurred, sleepy eyes, Anna's face slowly comes into focus.

                    ANNA (CONT'D)
          Girl, you look like you've been
          trying to ride a Denver bronco
          through a Texas twister.

Sarah tries to spring out from under her bed covers...

                    SARAH
          My boys!

Anna grabs her arm...

                    ANNA
          Easy. Easy. The boys are fine.
          They're playing in their room with
          Donovan.

Sarah plants her face into her hands, then rubs the morning from her eyes in order to focus.

                    SARAH
          Anna, you scared me to death.

                    ANNA
          Well how was I to know you'd be
          wound tight as a tetherball? What's
          up with you, girl?

                    SARAH
          Oh, just everything that's been
          going on with Eli.

Sarah glances at her alarm clock...

                    SARAH (CONT'D)
          And why are you in my bedroom at
          7:32 in the morning?

                    ANNA
          Can I not spend some quality time
          with my best friend? And Donovan
          wanted to bring the boys some
          belated gifts and candy for
          Valentine's Day.

Anna flops back on the bed, striking a sexy pose...

                    ANNA (CONT'D)
          Speaking of Valentine's Day, did
          you and Matthew have a... romantic
          evening together?

                    SARAH
          Oh, would you hush.

Sarah hops out of bed, staggering to the bathroom. Anna
unravels her pose, rolling over on the bed...

                    ANNA
          Just curious...

64   BATHROOM

Sarah gazes into the mirror, massaging her puffy eyes...

                    SARAH
          Well you better get un-curious,
          because I don't kiss and tell.

                    ANNA (O.S.)
          Just remember, he and Spense are
          best buds.

Sarah peeks her head into the bedroom, giving a, "You
wouldn't dare!" look.

                    ANNA (CONT'D)
          I'll find out one way or another.

65   BATHROOM

Sarah brushes her hair back into a ponytail...

                    SARAH
          We didn't even get to go out.

64

                    ANNA (O.S.)
          On Valentine's Day?

                    SARAH
          He was on call, and well, poor
          little Eli has just been so sick.

66   BEDROOM

Sarah goes back to the bed, pointing to her make-up-less face
and ponytail...

                    SARAH
          This is as good as it's gonna get
          today.

DONOVAN, now six-years-old, and NOAH come running into the
bedroom. DONOVAN has a Valentine's Day balloon on a string,
and NOAH has a stuffed teddy bear.

DONOVAN comes crashing onto Anna as she lies on the bed.

                    ANNA
               (winded)
          Holy cow... you're getting too big
          for that, son.

Noah runs over to Sarah...

                    NOAH
          Mommy, look what Donovan brought
          me.

Sarah grabs the teddy...

                    SARAH
          Have you given him a name yet?

                    NOAH
          Not yet, but I was thinking about
          calling him, Fluffy.

                    SARAH
          Well that would be a good name.
          Where's little brother?

                    NOAH
          He's in our bedroom. Hey, Mom, why
          does Eli look so sad today?

Sarah glances over at Anna with concern...

                    SARAH
          What do you mean?

Noah places his hand over the right side of his face...

                    NOAH
          This side of his face looks sad.

Sarah and Anna leap from the bed.

67   ELI'S BEDROOM

SARAH and ANNA come rushing in, finding ELI playing with his
stuffed doggy.

Sarah quickly examines him, finding the right side of his
face is drooping...

                    SARAH
          Honey, are you okay?

                    ELI
          Pretty good.

Sarah holds her left hand up to the right side of Eli's
head...

                    SARAH
          Eli, baby, can you see mommy's hand
          beside your head?

He shakes his head, no.

Sarah grabs up Eli and jets passed Anna, down the hallway to
the living room. Anna follows close behind.

68   LIVING ROOM

                    SARAH
          Can you stay here with Noah?

                    ANNA
          Of course.

                    ANNA (CONT'D)
          What's going on?

Still in her pj's, Sarah grabs her purse, rushing to the
door...

                    SARAH
          No time. I'll call you from the ER.

69   INT. DURANGO HOSPITAL- LATER

SARAH sits on an examination table in her pj's, holding Eli.

DR. OWENS and DR. JAMES stand before her.

                    SARAH
          Please. Please tell me you've
          figured it out. Tell me you've got
          something.

                    DR. OWENS
          Well, we've determined that it
          wasn't a stroke that has caused the
          side of your son's face to droop
          like it is.

Sarah shows slight relief.

                    DR. JAMES
          It's possible that your son might
          have Bells Palsy, but I'm not
          certain.

                    DR. OWENS
          Look... Sarah... we don't know if
          we've missed something along the
          way, so we've scheduled another CT
          scan for Eli at Frisco, in
          Silverthorne.

                    DR. JAMES
          Mrs. Logan, rest assured, we will
          get to the bottom of this.

70   EXT. SARAH'S APARTMENT- SAME DAY

SARAH pulls into the parking lot. Just before retrieving Eli
from the car, she hears two truck doors slamming across the
way. She turns to find both ETHER and HENRY speed-walking
toward her.

Henry blows up.

                    HENRY
          Where's my boy?

Sarah places her hand in the middle of Henry's chest,
stopping his progress to Eli...

                    SARAH
          What's going on here?

                    HENRY
        I said, "Where's my boy?"

Henry goes to grab Sarah as she slaps his hands away...

                    SARAH
        Touch me and you'll be spending the
        next six months in the County.
              (to Ethel)
        The same goes for you, Mother.

Henry jabs his finger at Sarah's face...

                    HENRY
        Those are my boys.

                    ETHEL JACKSON
        And they're my grandchildren.

                    ANNA
        Grandchildren!

Anna closes the apartment door behind her as she swaggers her
way onto the scene.

                    ANNA (CONT'D)
        Shouldn't a lady first learn how to
        become a mother, before ever trying
        to be a grandmother?
              (to Henry)
        And you. If you ever want to be a
        daddy to these boys, then you'd
        better start by showing their
        mother some respect.

Anna turns and winks at Sarah...

                    ANNA (CONT'D)
        Get Eli inside.

                    HENRY
              (to Anna)
        You've got no right--

                    ANNA
        Rights?

Anna almost bodies-up to Henry...

> ANNA (CONT'D)
> With every medical record of
> Sarah's that I've kept over the
> years - and I've got'em all - I can
> take away every right that you
> *think* you still have.

Sarah whisks Eli into the apartment, as Henry tries his
finger-jab at Anna's face.

> HENRY
> Now you listen to me--

Anna grabs Henry's finger, focusing on its tip...

> ANNA
> You ever see what a Ball-peen
> hammer can do to the tips of
> someone's fingers?

Henry jerks his hand away.

> ANNA (CONT'D)
> I know a very, very big Italian man
> who is just dying to show you.

Ethel and Henry look at one another.

> ANNA (CONT'D)
> Look. If you two are hoping to have
> any time with those precious boys
> in the near future, then I suggest
> you start acting like adults. But I
> can assure you, there will be no
> more of this nonsense; not while
> I'm around.

> ETHEL JACKSON
> Let's go Henry. It's easy to see
> when you're not wanted.

71   INT. FRISCO HOSPITAL- DAY

SUPERIMPOSE:
> Frisco Hospital, March
> 5th, 1990

It's the wee hours of the morning. In the waiting room, an
exhausted looking SARAH clings tightly around MATTHEW'S neck.

> SARAH
> Thank you so much for stopping by.

Matthew squeezes even tighter around her waist.

                    MATTHEW
          You know it's my pleasure, Sarah.

Releasing the tension of the hug, they gaze upon one another.

                    MATTHEW (CONT'D)
          Is there anything else I can do for
          you: bring you breakfast, a change
          of clothes... anything?

                    SARAH
          Just waiting on the results from
          Eli's scans. Thanks, but I have
          both of my boys here with me... and
          right now that's all I need.

                    MATTHEW
          Well, you know I'm available. Just
          call my pager if you need anything
          at all.

                    SARAH
          You know I will.

72   INT. FRISCO HOSPITAL- LATER

In the hospital room, Eli lays asleep in the bed. SARAH sits
next to him in a comfortable reclining chair, holding a
sleeping Noah in her arms.

DR. BROWN (mid-50s), somewhat short and a little overweight,
enters the room with DR. NOONAN (mid-40s), tall and slender.

                    DR. BROWN
          Good morning Mrs. Logan. I'm Dr.
          Brown, the Pediatrics Specialist
          here at Frisco... and of course you
          know Dr. Noonan, who performed the
          procedure a while back of placing
          tubes into Eli's ears.

Dr. Brown motions toward the hallway...

                    Dr. BROWN (CONT'D)
          May we speak to you for a moment?

Sarah slowly stands, gently placing a sleeping Noah back down
into the chair.

73   HALLWAY

                              SARAH
                    Did the scans tell us anything?

The doctors glance at one another.

                              DR. NOONAN
                    Mrs. Logan, while going over the
                    scans with the radiologist... I'm
                    sorry to say, but we've found that
                    there is a soft tissue mass-a
                    pharyngeal tumor extending up
                    through the cerebral fossa and into
                    Eli's brain cavity.

Stunned, Sarah falls back against the wall.

Dr. Brown places his hand on her shoulder...

                              DR. BROWN
                    Mrs. Logan... Sarah, Dr. Noonan
                    will still need to do a biopsy in
                    order to make a proper diagnosis.
                    So until then, there is no need to
                    panic. Afterwards, we'll need to
                    get him to the University Hospital
                    in Denver for treatments.

                              DR. NOONAN
                    He is correct, Sarah. Let us first
                    determine what the tissue is, then
                    we can begin our attack against it.

Sarah replies with a dazed nod of the head.

                              DR. BROWN
                    Until then, should you need
                    anything, Dr. Noonan and I will be
                    around to assist you or answer any
                    questions you might have.

                              DR. NOONAN
                    We'll talk soon Mrs. Logan.

As the doctors leave, still in a fog, Sarah slowly makes her
way to the end of the hallway, staring out the window.

She looks to the sky and pleads through tears...

                              SARAH
                    How selfish can you be? One isn't
                    enough? You stay away from my son.

FLASH FORWARD

74   INT. UNIVERSITY OF COLORADO HOSPITAL- NIGHT 1990

The hand of a thirty-year-old woman writes in a journal that
rests on her lap. Numerous Kleenex tissues surround her,
scattered across what appears to be the seat cushion of a
pew.

                    YOUNG ADULT FEMALE (V.O.)
               Little Eli was diagnosed with
               Rhabdomyosarcoma; a soft tissue
               cancer that had originated in his
               neck. Her baby boy had already
               suffered so much, but nothing could
               have prepared them for the road
               ahead.

75   EXT. UNIVERSITY OF COLORADO HOSPITAL- DAY

SUPERIMPOSE:

     University of Colorado Hospital- Denver, CO.

               ONE MONTH LATER

It's early morning. SARAH and ELI lay asleep, cuddled
together in the hospital bed.

The phone rings. Sarah jumps to answer it before Eli awakens.

                    SARAH
               (into phone)
          Hello.
               (listening)

Sarah's countenance brightens...

                    SARAH (CONT'D)
               (into phone)
          And good morning to you too. How's
          momma's big boy?
               (listening)
          An A+? I'm so proud of you, Noah. I
          wish I could--
               (listening)
          Oh, well you'd better hurry then.
          You have a great day at school...
          and mommy loves you.

Sarah hangs up the phone, picking up her daily journal that
lays on the night stand.

She flips through it until finding the date...

> SARAH (CONT'D)
> Three weeks... already?

Her focus draws to Eli, as a huge smile appears on her face. She sneaks over to seize the precious moment of watching him sleep.

With his head wrapped in a bandage from the surgery, Sarah runs her fingertips through his hair atop his head- just above the gauze wrap. Her smile slowly evaporates, replaced by an expression of a harsh reality. She draws her hand near her face, finding it full of Eli's golden locks of hair.

Sarah quickly removes the loose hair from Eli's pillow, throwing it into a nearby trash can. Turning around, she is surprised to find Ethel standing in the doorway.

> SARAH (CONT'D)
> Mother, you scared me.

> ETHEL JACKSON
> (hateful)
> Would you just look at my grandson?
> You are a worthless mother.

> SARAH
> Ethel--

> ETHEL JACKSON
> Uh. Uh. Uh.

Ethel retrieves a tiny recorder from her purse.

> ETHEL JACKSON (CONT'D)
> Now, I'll have proof of what a
> miserable excuse you are.

Sarah brushes by Ethel and leans into the hallway...

> SARAH
> (yelling)
> Nurse. I need security.

Sarah steps back into the room.

> SARAH (CONT'D)
> Ethel, get out.

Ethel waves the recorder in Sarah's face...

> ETHEL JACKSON
> I have a right to visit my
> grandson.

Eli awakens with groggy tears from the shouting.

> ELI
> Make her leave, Mommy. Make her
> leave.

> ETHEL JACKSON
> Now look what you've done.

> SARAH
> What I've done? Get out!

Security rushes in, removing Ethel as she lashes out to Sarah.

Sarah rushes to comfort Eli.

> SARAH (CONT'D)
> It's okay, Eli. Mommy's here.
> Everything's going to be just fine.

76   INT. UNIVERSITY OF COLORADO HOSPITAL- DAY

By the handles on his wheelchair, SARAH vrooms ELI into his hospital room as though he's driving a race car. ELI is sporting racing goggles just below the gauze on his head, acting as though he's gripping a steering wheel.

SARAH brings the make-shift roadster to a screeching halt beside his bed.

> SARAH
> Err... time for a nap Speed Racer.

Eli hops onto the bed as Sarah tucks him in.

> ELI
> Can we do it again tomorrow, Mommy?

> SARAH
> I don't know... you think we can
> set a new land-speed record?

> ELI
> Yeah!

Sarah leans down for a kiss.

74

                    SARAH
          We'll see, munchkin.

Sarah begins folding some clothes that lay on the empty bed
in the room.

Eli springs up from the pillow, pawing at the bandage on his
head...

                    ELI
          Mom! My head don't hurt no more.

He then rubs his neck...

                    ELI (CONT'D)
          Mom! My neck don't hurt no more.

Sarah rushes to his bedside, blinking back the tears.

                    SARAH
          That's good son.

                    ELI
          Mom, sometimes when I got up in the
          night and went to your bed, I was
          not scared. I just had a big head
          hurt.

                    SARAH
          Son, why didn't you ever tell me?

                    ELI
          It don't hurt no more, Mommy.

Sarah hugs him tightly.

                    SARAH
          We're going to make it, little man.
          We're going to make it.

77   INT. UNIVERSITY OF COLORADO HOSPITAL- DAY

SARAH is tidying up the hospital room and straightening the
covers on Eli's bed.

SARAH calls out to ELI in the bathroom...

                    SARAH
          Don't worry, sweetie, you've got
          plenty of time.

                    ELI (O.S.)
          Okay, Mom.

The phone rings. Sarah answers cheerfully...

>   SARAH
>   (into phone)
>   Good morning, Momma's big man.
>   (listening)

She rolls her eyes in disgust...

>   SARAH (CONT'D)
>   What do you need Henry?
>   (listening)
>   Don't be disgusting.
>   (listening)
>   Well you'll have to hold on a
>   minute; he's in the bathroom.
>   (listening)
>   I'm not lying--

As Henry begins screaming into the phone, Sarah pulls it away
from her ear, before nonchalantly hanging up on him.

>   ELI (O.C.)
>   Who was that, Mommy?

Eli rolls into the room in his wheelchair, with noticeably
less hair than he once had. The drooping of the right side of
his face is more noticeable, as he speaks through the left
side of his mouth.

>   SARAH
>   Oh... Hey sweetie. Well I could
>   think of several things to call
>   him, but I'd rather...

She picks up a bag and pulls out a stuffed animal.

>   SARAH (CONT'D)
>   ...give you a birthday present.

Eli smiles, grabbing the animal and hugging it tightly, as
Sarah leans over to hug Eli tightly.

>   SARAH (CONT'D)
>   I can't believe my little man is
>   already five-years-old.

>   ELI
>   Mommy, since it's my birthday, do
>   we have to go today?

Sarah kneels down before him...

                     SARAH
Eli, Honey, do you know that I'd do
anything for you to not have to be
here?

                     ELI
Would you even go to the moon and
back?

                     SARAH
I'd even go to the moon and back.

                     ELI
Would you even eat those green peas
that you don't like.

Sarah grimaces, before proudly raising her chin high...

                     SARAH
I'd eat a whole mountain of those
green peas. But right now, it's
this radiation stuff that is
helping to make you better.

                     ELI
Is it killing the cancer ghosts?

                     SARAH
        (smiling)
That's exactly right. And who
knows, today might be better than
last time.

She grabs the handles and wheels him out of the room.

78   INT. UNIVERSITY OF COLORADO HOSPITAL- LATER

SARAH wheels ELI toward radiation oncology. As they approach
the room, they find Eli's nurse, NURSE VICKI (mid-40s),
standing in the hallway, with the door to the room closed
behind her.

                  NURSE VICKI
        (to Eli)
Well what do we have here?

Nurse Vicki gives the stuffed animal a pat on the head.

                     ELI
It's my birthday, Nurse Vicki.

                         NURSE VICKI
          Well, if we'd known, maybe we could
          have planned something for you.

She gives Sarah a wink.

                    NURSE VICKI (CONT'D)
                    (to Eli)
          Are you ready to get rid of some
          more of those cancer ghosts?

Eli gives a cheerful nod.

The nurse opens the door to the room.

79   ONCOLOGY ROOM

       Eli is greeted with a resounding, "Surprise!", from a room
       full of nurses, radiation technicians and others.

       Through the pain of the drooping right side of his face and
       the treatments, Eli musters the biggest smile imaginable, as
       Sarah wheels him into the room. The nurses are snapping
       Polaroid's as he sees a huge banner that reads, "Happy
       Birthday Eli."

       The radiation table is decorated with balloons, and is
       overflowing with toys.

       Sarah leans down, whispering into Eli's ear and pointing
       toward the back of the room.

       It's Anna and Noah. Anna releases Noah, as he sprints to give
       his baby brother a hug. Anna then embraces Sarah.

       Amid the celebration, the room is quickly silenced as JOEY
       (6), a tiny bald-headed boy wearing a patients gown, breaks
       free from his mother's side, confidently approaching Eli and
       handing him a heart-shaped pillow.

                         JOEY
          Happy birthday, Eli.

       Eli, taken back, reaches up to feel what little of his own
       hair he has left.

       Sarah kneels to Eli's side, pulling his hand away from his
       head...

                         SARAH
          It's okay, son.

                         JOEY
          Yeah, now you're almost like me...
          You're almost like all of us.

Joey turns and points, as about a dozen parents stand beside
each of their tiny, bald-headed children.

Joey leans toward Eli, offering up his bald head.

                         JOEY (CONT'D)
          See... feel.

Eli looks to his mother for affirmation.

                         SARAH
          It's okay.

Rubbing Joey's head, The left side of Eli's mouth turns up in
a smile.

Joey leans in even closer to Eli...

                         JOEY
                   (whispering)
          And we never have to wash our hair.

                         NURSE VICKI
          Eli, are you ready to open some
          birthday presents?

                         ELI
          Yeah!

80   INT. UNIVERSITY OF COLORADO HOSPITAL- DAY

       There is a tiny, almost bald head, as Sarah snips the last
       strand of Eli's hair with a pair of scissors. There are
       several tiny bald-heads in Eli's room at the time, all giving
       cheer at the final snip.

81   INT. UNIVERSITY OF COLORADO HOSPITAL- DAY

       Eli, Noah and Joey are running around a nurses station, each
       hiding behind nurses and doctors as they are having a squirt-
       gun war.

82   INT. UNIVERSITY OF COLORADO HOSPITAL- NIGHT

       Sarah and Eli lay in bed, each wearing a surgical mask as she
       reads him a Dr. Seuss book.

83   INT. UNIVERSITY OF COLORADO HOSPITAL- NIGHT

      While Eli sits up in bed, Sarah holds a plastic trash-can
      steady, catching his vomit.

84   INT. UNIVERSITY OF COLORADO HOSPITAL- NIGHT

      In a hallway of the hospital, Henry stands face to face with
      Sarah, lashing out at her. Hospital security rushes in,
      dragging Henry away as he continues his rant.

85   INT. SARAH'S APARTMENT- NIGHT

      Hannah and Noah sit cuddled together on the couch in a dimly
      lit living room. She is reading him a letter.

      ONSCREEN

      Atop the letter reads: To Noah, From Mommy and Brother.

86   INT. UNIVERSITY OF COLORADO HOSPITAL- NIGHT

      As Eli lay asleep in his bed, under a night stand in the
      corner of the room Sarah opens a Hallmark card addressed to
      her.

      ONSCREEN

      "To the best mother in the world! Happy Mother's Day!
      Matthew..."

      SARAH

      Draws the card near to her heart and smiles.

87   INT. UNIVERSITY OF COLORADO HOSPITAL- NIGHT

      Eli is sitting up in his bed. With a mother's concern, Sarah
      holds a plastic trash-can as Eli is vomiting into it.

88   INT. UNIVERSITY OF COLORADO HOSPITAL- DAY

      Eli and Joey are playing Super Mario on the Nintendo in Eli's
      room.

89   INT. UNIVERSITY OF COLORADO HOSPITAL- NIGHT

In his dimly lit room, Sarah sits in a recliner next to Eli,
watching him as he sleeps. With her knees cuddled to her
chest, she sobs into a pillow.

90   INT. UNIVERSITY OF COLORADO HOSPITAL- DAY

SARAH pushes ELI in a wheelchair where they visit the
classroom, the nurses station, the medication room, and
finally the newborn nursery.

Eli says with a weak voice...

                    ELI
          Mommy, I want to take the babies
          with me when we get to go back
          home.

                    SARAH
          Oh, sweetie. Babies have to go home
          with *their* mommies.

Eli smiles. Sarah continues pushing the wheelchair down the
hallway.

END MONTAGE

91   INT. UNIVERSITY OF COLORADO HOSPITAL- DAY

BLACK SCREEN.

                    NURSE VICKI (O.S.)
               (whispering)
          Mrs. Logan... Mrs. Logan.

It is early in the morning. NURSE VICKI is trying to awaken
SARAH as she lays asleep in the recliner next to Eli's bed.

Sarah jumps in fear...

                    SARAH
          What's wrong!?

                    NURSE VICKI
          Eli is fine, Sarah.

They both glance over to find him peacefully sleeping.

                    NURSE VICKI (CONT'D)
          Could I speak to you outside?

92   HALLWAY

                         SARAH
               Is everything okay?

Nurse Vicki grabs Sarah's hands, trying to calm her nerves.

                         NURSE VICKI
               Sarah, nothing has changed with
               Eli. I just... I just knew that Eli
               and Joey were going to watch the
               fireworks display together tonight.

Sarah finally exhales...

                         SARAH
               Oh, yes, of course. You had me
               startled. I can't believe it's
               already July.

Sarah rubs the sleep from her eyes...

                         SARAH (CONT'D)
               So what happened... did they cancel
               the display?

                         NURSE VICKI
               This is never easy.
                    (beat)
               Sarah, little Joey went home last
               night.

                         SARAH
               Well good for him. Did his mother
               happen to leave any contact infor--

                         NURSE VICKI
               Mrs. Logan, he went home to be with
               the Lord.

                         SARAH
               Oh my...

Sarah flinches, momentarily standing in a daze.

                         SARAH (CONT'D)
               Uh, well... I'll uh...

She motions to the door of Eli's room, then quietly enters,
closing the door behind her.

93   INT. UNIVERSITY OF COLORADO HOSPITAL- NIGHT

        Sarah is kicked back in the recliner, clinging to Eli. The
        two of them stare somewhat emotionless out the window of
        Eli's hospital room, watching, as the fireworks explode into
        all different colors.

94   INT. UNIVERSITY OF COLORADO HOSPITAL- DAY

        SUPERIMPOSE:
                        JULY 19TH, 1990

        Sarah has a huge smile as she looks down.

                            SARAH
                Eli. Eli, honey.

        She shakes her son ever so gently to awaken him.

        As he comes too, he sees his mother, along with Nurse Vicki
        and several other doctors and nurses standing over him.

                            SARAH (CONT'D)
                Guess what?

        Eli preciously grins...

                            ELI
                Are we going home?

                            SARAH
                We're going home!

        The nurses throw confetti as everyone cheers.

95   INT. UNIVERSITY OF COLORADO HOSPITAL- LATER

        With suitcases packed and sitting atop the gurney in Eli's
        room, SARAH and ELI await patiently for his release.

        SARAH is sitting in the recliner, writing in her journal, as
        ELI sits in a wheelchair with his arms wrapped tightly around
        Donatello - a giant, stuffed Teenage Mutant Ninja Turtle.

        NURSE VICKI enters with DR. MORAN (MID 50S), tall and clean
        cut.

                            NURSE VICKI
                Mrs. Logan, this is Dr. Moran. He
                will be overseeing the results of
                the recent CT scans.

The doctor extends his hand...

                    DR. MORAN
        Pleasure to meet you Mrs. Logan...
        and you as well, Eli.
            (to Sarah)
        Look, I don't need to remind you of
        all that you've experienced over
        the past several months. We may or
        may not be in the clear, but...

The doctor holds up a manila folder.

                    DR. MORAN (CONT'D)
        ...I have the scans from yesterday.
        We'll call you with results as soon
        as we know something; hopefully no
        longer than a few days.

                    SARAH
        Sounds good.

                    DR. MORAN
        I know it's easier said than done,
        but try not to think about it. You
        two have a safe trip home, and
        we'll talk soon.

The doctor leans down, shaking Eli's hand...

                    DR. MORAN (CONT'D)
        You're an incredibly brave young
        man, Eli. Will you look after
        Leonardo for me?

Eli squeezes the stuffed turtle tightly...

                    ELI
        It's Donatello.

                    DR. MORAN
        I stand corrected.

                    SARAH
            (to doctor)
        Are we free?

                    DR. MORAN
        Mrs. Logan, you are free to go.

96   INT. SARAH'S APARTMENT- DAY

SARAH and ANNA sit at the kitchen table, drinking coffee as
they watch Donovan, Eli and Noah playing with toy cars in the
living room floor.

                    SARAH
          I'm so glad you guys dropped in.

                    ANNA
          Are you kidding? Donovan couldn't
          wait to get here. And I hear Eli's
          story is going to be in the
          newspaper?

Sarah smiles while watching the boys...

                    SARAH
          So proud of that little guy. He and
          Noah have barely slept a wink in
          the few days we've been back.

Sarah's smile fades into a look of sorrow. Anna tries to
cheer her up...

                    ANNA
          So let me get this straight: You're
          back home with the boys, you've got
          a new man, and Donovan said that
          "Make a Wish" is sending you guys
          to Disneyland...? I bet the kids
          are so excited.

Sarah gives a dazed nod.

                    ANNA (CONT'D)
          Why do I get the feeling there is a
          "but" coming? It's not Matt is it?
          Is he being a jerk, because--

                    SARAH
          "But," we have to go back.

                    ANNA
               (remorseful)
          Oh, Sarah... do the kids--

                    SARAH
          No. I just don't have the heart.
          They called yesterday, saying the
          scans show a large mass in his
          right lung.

                    ANNA
          Poor little guy.

                    SARAH
          He's just so weak, Anna.

Sarah blinks back the tears.

                    SARAH (CONT'D)
          I just don't know how much more his
          little body can take.

97   INT. SARAH'S APARTMENT- NIGHT

Sarah lays between NOAH and ELI in bed, all three are asleep.
The silence of the night is broken when Noah awakens.

Noah cries out as though his little brother is lost...

                    NOAH
          Brother! Brother!

Eli is stirred, hops out of bed, runs around to the other
side. Meeting Noah with a huge bear-hug.

                    ELI
          I'm right here, Bubbie.

Sarah cherishes the moment.

98   EXT. SARAH'S APARTMENT- DAY

SARAH and ANNA finish loading the car for the trip back to
Denver. ELI sits in the front passenger seat.

                    ELI
          Mommy, did you bring Donatello?

                    SARAH
          You bet, sweetie.

MATTHEW slams the hood of the car, as SPENCER crawls out from
underneath, both covered in grease. NOAH stands off to the
side next to Hannah.

                    SPENCER
               (to Sarah)
          Well, we replaced the leaky oil pan
          gasket--

                    MATTHEW
          But, the compressor is shot.

                    SARAH
          So, no A/C?

                    MATTHEW
          Sorry. But, hey... why don't you
          just take my truck.

                    SARAH
          Aww, thanks. But I wouldn't have
          time to move everything over from
          the car.

Anna leans in for a hug.

                    ANNA
          Hey, we'll get it fixed when you
          get back. And I'll be up to see you
          in a couple of days.

                    SARAH
               (to everyone)
          Thanks guys... for all you've done
          for us.

Sarah leans down to hug Noah.

                    SARAH (CONT'D)
          Did you say goodbye to your
          brother?

Noah runs around the car to the passenger window, reaching in
and patting Eli's bald head.

                    NOAH
          I love you, Bubbie.

                    ELI
          I love you too, Noah.

Noah hands Eli a tiny object through the window.

                    NOAH
               (whispering)
          Take this. It'll protect you.

Sarah hugs Matthew.

                    SARAH
          Thanks again. I'll call you tonight
          after we get settled in.

Sarah jumps in the car and heads to Denver.

99   INT. UNIVERSITY OF COLORADO HOSPITAL- DAY

SUPERIMPOSED:
            JULY 31ST, 1990

In a holding room, ELI lays on a gurney while SARAH and a PRE-OP NURSE (30s), are busy getting him ready for surgery.

Eli holds Donatello in his arms.

                    ELI
            Mommy, why is there a cancer ghost
            in my chest?

Sarah places a scrub cap on his head.

                    SARAH
                (playful)
            It's just one more little cancer
            ghost that got left behind.

                    ELI
            And then I go to ICU?

                    PRE-OP NURSE
            What a very smart little boy, you
            are.

                    SARAH
            Yes he is. He starts kindergarten
            in the Fall.

Sarah leans down, kissing Eli's cheek.

                    SARAH (CONT'D)
            Yes. And then you go to ICU.

Eli grabs Sarah's face with both hands.

                    ELI
            Mommy, am I going to die?

Sarah and the nurse freeze, sharing a glance.

                    ELI (CONT'D)
            Am I going to go to Heaven where
            Joshua is?

Sarah deflects. Panicking, tucking him in snug.

                    SARAH
            Well... no. Why would you think
            such a thing? Mommy and brother
            need you here.

                         ELI
          I want to go to Heaven, Mom. I want
          to go to Heaven and Jesus.

With her back to Eli, Sarah's jaws clinch in anger, before
turning to him with a fake smile.

                         SARAH
          Son, we don't always get what we
          want in life. So you might just
          have to come back to me.

Sarah rubs the tip of his nose, playfully trying to lighten
the mood.

                         SARAH (CONT'D)
          Now you quit worrying so much.
          We'll be back home in no time.
          (beat) Mommy has to step out for a
          minute, but I'll be right back.

                         ELI
          Okay, Mommy.

100   HALLWAY

Sarah steps out of the room, collapsing against the wall in
tears. Down the way, she spots a doctor approaching a young
couple. With a loud shriek, the young mother's knees buckle
as she crumbles into his arms.

101   INT. UNIVERSITY OF COLORADO HOSPITAL- NIGHT 1990

The hand of a thirty-year-old woman writes in the journal
that rests upon her lap. Next to her, on what appears to be a
pew, is several scattered used Kleenex tissues.

                         YOUNG ADULT FEMALE (V.O.)
               (sniffling)
          Her heart was broken. How could Her
          baby boy have known so much of
          Heaven, though she had refused to
          speak of it?

The writing hand pauses. As the journal in her lap slowly
draws nearer and nearer, her hand continues to pen the story.

                         YOUNG ADULT FEMALE (V.O.)
          How selfish she had been--

                         ANNA (O.C.)
          Sarah...?

The hand stops writing.

ANNA stands in the doorway, stunned to find Sarah sitting in the middle of the front row pew of the hospital chapel.

Sarah silently looks over her shoulder, grieving, before turning back to hide her face in her hands.

Anna slowly approaches.

                    ANNA (CONT'D)
          Sarah. Are you okay, honey?

Anna places her arm around Sarah while sliding in next to her.

Sarah finally gains enough composure to speak.

                    SARAH
          I bet this is the last place you
          thought you'd find me?

                    ANNA
          Well...

                    SARAH
          I asked the nurse not to bother me
          unless it was important.

                    ANNA
          They said Eli did very well.

                    SARAH
          Yeah. He's a trooper. (beat) He's
          sleeping right now, so I thought
          I'd take a few minutes to myself. I
          just dread the radiation again.
          He's so much stronger than I could
          ever be. From day one he's stood up
          and fought this thing.

                    ANNA
          I don't know... sounds a lot like
          his momma.

Sarah ashamedly shakes her head.

                    SARAH
          You know what I realized today,
          Anna? I realized that I have spent
          my entire life running. First it
          was from Ethel, and then from
          Henry.

                    ANNA
          As would anyone in their right
          mind.

                    SARAH
          But that's just it. It's not about
          who I was running *from*. It's the
          fact that I've spent my entire life
          chasing after some... fairy-tale.

Sarah holds up her journal.

                    SARAH (CONT'D)
          Even when I write, I pretend I'm
          not the one who actually had to
          live out this Godforsaken
          nightmare; like I'm on the outside
          looking in. (beat) The day I
          married Henry, I made a promise to
          God... that if He'd give me
          children, I'd become a mother that
          He'd be proud of.

                    ANNA
          And you have...

Sarah lets out a guilty chuckle.

                    SARAH
          Anna, when I left Silverthorne, I
          wasn't running from Henry anymore.

A wrinkle of confusion emerges between Anna's eyes.

                    SARAH (CONT'D)
          I was running from God.

                    ANNA
               (lovingly)
          We've all been guilty of that,
          Sarah.

                    SARAH
          You don't understand. After my...
          after Joshua, I tried. But I had
          become so bitter; so angry. And now
          I feel so ashamed. (beat) Today my
          son told me that he was ready to go
          to Heaven... and I've spent his
          entire life trying to keep him away
          from it.

Sarah falls over into Anna's arms. Sobbing.

Sarah shrieks...

> SARAH (CONT'D)
> ...I never told him.

102   INT. UNIVERSITY OF COLORADO HOSPITAL- DAY

SARAH and DR. MORAN stand in the hallway just outside of
Eli's room.

Sarah is gitty.

> DR. MORAN
> Radiation has been going well, Mrs.
> Logan, but let me remind you that
> it's only been a few weeks since
> his surgery. Therefore--

> SARAH
> Be careful... got it.

> DR. MORAN
> Just be mindful of the fact.

> SARAH
> Thank you so much Dr. Moran.

103   ELI'S ROOM

SARAH excitedly makes her way over, sitting on the bed next
to a very weak ELI as he is watching television.

> SARAH
> What do you say we sneak out of
> here today and go have some fun?

> ELI
> Like what, Mommy?

> SARAH
> Oh, I don't know. I guess you'll
> just have to wait and see.

104   I/E. SARAH'S CAR- DAY

SARAH and ELI sit inside her parked car. ELI, wearing a
baseball cap, is covering his eyes with both hands.

> SARAH
> Alright, no peeking.

>   ELI
>   I won't, Mommy.

Sarah hops out, and is met at the trunk of her car by a
Denver Zoo employee, male (20s), who gives her a zoo
stroller.

She rushes, opening the passenger door of the car.

>   SARAH
>   Did I see you peek?

>   ELI
>   No, Mommy. I promise.

She lifts Eli from the car, placing him into the stroller.

Sarah turns the stroller around to the entrance of the zoo.

>   SARAH
>   Okay. You can look.

>   ELI
>   The zoo!

105   I/E. DENVER ZOO- DAY

Sarah takes pictures as ELI rides a Shetland pony.

>   ELI
>   Just like a real cowboy, Mommy.

106   I/E. DENVER ZOO- DAY

SARAH and ELI are glaring at huge turtles.

Eli excitedly points...

>   ELI
>   That one looks like Donatello.

>   SARAH
>   He does...?

107   I/E. DENVER ZOO- DAY

From his stroller, Eli is taking a picture of Sarah, who
squeamishly stands in front of a tiger's cage.

108   I/E. DENVER ZOO- DAY

       SARAH is pushing ELI in the stroller, approaching the exit.

                         SARAH
                 Was that fun or what?

                         ELI
                 Yep. But I'm getting hot, Mommy.

                         SARAH
                 Well let me see if I can help you
                 cool off a bit.

       Sarah takes off Eli's hat, using it to fan his face.

       A ZOO EMPLOYEE, female (20-ish), approaches...

                         ZOO EMPLOYEE
                 May I help you with the stroller,
                 ma'am?

                         SARAH
                 You bet. Just cooling him down real
                 quick.

       A YOUNG BOY (12-ish) is walking by with his classmates.

       He looks at Eli...

                         YOUNG BOY
                   (to classmates)
                 Look everybody. Run! It's an alien.

       Though enraged that Eli heard the statement, Sarah gently
       places the cap back on his head, lifts him from the stroller
       and walks away.

                         SARAH
                   (to Eli)
                 So what did you think about those
                 Giraffe's long necks...?

                         ELI
                 They were neat, Mommy.

109   INT. UNIVERSITY OF COLORADO HOSPITAL- NIGHT

       Asleep on her shoulder, SARAH carries ELI to his hospital
       room. While removing his cap, he awakens as she tucks him in.

>   SARAH
>   I have to step out for just a
>   second, my love, but I'll be right
>   back.

Leaning down, she kisses him on the head.

>   ELI
>   I'm sorry, mommy.

>   SARAH
>   Why?

>   ELI
>   I'm sorry, mommy.

>   SARAH
>   Eli, for what?

>   ELI
>   I'm sorry that I want to go home.

>   SARAH
>   Oh, Hun. We'll go home as soon as
>   we possibly can.

She gives him another kiss on the head.

>   SARAH (CONT'D)
>   I'll be right back.

As she leaves, Eli reaches beneath his pillow, pulls out a
tiny object his brother had given him, kisses it, and places
it back under the pillow.

110   HALLWAY

Closing the door behind her, Sarah has a puzzled, almost
fearful countenance.

>   SARAH (V.O.)
>   Eli always had a way with words;
>   causing me to stop and face
>   reality. At that moment, I couldn't
>   help but think the home he was
>   referring to was heaven.

111   INT. UNIVERSITY OF COLORADO HOSPITAL- DAY

ELI lays in pain, silently crying. Cold sores and blisters
all around his mouth and lips. SARAH sits in a bedside chair
trying to comfort him.

> SARAH
> I know, Eli. I'm so sorry, my love.

She places her hand upon his brow.

> SARAH (CONT'D)
> You're burning up.

> ELI
> Mommy, can I go back to the room
> that kills the cancer ghosts?

> SARAH
> Oh, son. We can't do radiation
> right now.

DR. MORAN enters the room. Sarah greets him at the door for private conversation.

> DR. MORAN
> Mrs. Logan, has Eli ever had the
> chickenpox?

> SARAH
> When he was two. Is this shingles?

> DR. MORAN
> It's difficult to say. But we do
> know it's some form of a herpes
> outbreak.

Sarah's jaws clinch.

> SARAH
> I'm so sick of this. Can it be
> treated?

> DR. MORAN
> Yes. We'll have to put him on an
> anti-viral drip for the next seven
> to ten days. But following that,
> he'll have to finish his treatment
> with a hard five-day chemo series.

Sarah looks back at Eli with despair.

112   INT. UNIVERSITY OF COLORADO HOSPITAL- NIGHT

SARAH is down on both knees at the front of the hospital chapel. With palms on the floor, she looks up at the cross that hangs on the wall directly in front of the room.

Emotional.

                    SARAH
               (to the cross)
          I am so angry. I'm so mad at you
          right now. Will you please...

She lashes out.

                    SARAH (CONT'D)
          Help. My. Son.

She slouches back on her heels. Weeping.

                    SARAH (CONT'D)
          If I've done something... punish
          me.

Leaning forward, with clinched fists she repeatedly bangs her
hands on the floor.

                    SARAH (CONT'D)
          He's done nothing wrong. He's just
          a child.

She stares at the floor with closed eyes.

                    SARAH (CONT'D)
               (quietly)
          How can you just sit back...

In a moment of clarity she rocks back on her heels once
again, brushes the hair from her face, and opens her eyes,
fixing them upon the Jesus who hangs on the cross before her.

                    SARAH (CONT'D)
          ...And watch him suffer?

Sarah rushes out of the room.

113   INT. UNIVERSITY OF COLORADO HOSPITAL- DAY

Eli's room is full of smiling nurses and doctors. Sarah
stands next to Eli's bed, along with Father Jacobs, who is
baptizing him.

                    SARAH (V.O.)
          Shortly thereafter, Eli was
          baptized by Father Jacobs. He
          received the sacrament, along with
          the anointing of the sick.

114   INT. DURANGO COLORADO- DAY

Hannah and Noah sit amid a congregation in a Catholic church.

                    SARAH (V.O.)
          Though Henry was furious, I
          informed him that, in my absence,
          Hannah would be taking Noah to
          church on Saturday evenings. If I
          could do nothing else, that was one
          wrong I was going to make right.

115   INT. UNIVERSITY OF COLORADO HOSPITAL- NIGHT

Superimpose:
          September 30th, 1990

SARAH sits bedside, reading Dr. Seuss to a very weak Eli.
NURSE VICKI enters the room, gently placing the back of her
hand on Eli's forehead, checking for a temperature.

                    NURSE VICKI
          How's our big man doing?

Sarah closes the book...

                    SARAH
          Still fighting that fever. And he's
          really going through the platelets.

Eli slowly raises his hand that loosely grips a squirt-gun.
Nurse Vicki holds her hands up...

                    NURSE VICKI
          You caught me Sheriff.

Eli tries to squeeze the trigger. His hand is too weak as it
falls back to the bed.

Nurse Vicki glances at the helplessness in Sarah's
countenance.

                    NURSE VICKI (CONT'D)
                 (to Eli)
          Looks like someone's tired. Eli,
          you get a good nights rest for your
          mother. Can you do that?

Eli gives a weak nod. Nurse Vicki gives Sarah a look of
sympathy before leaving.

116   INT. UNIVERSITY OF COLORADO HOSPITAL- DAY

        SUPERIMPOSE:
                    October 1st, 1990

        SARAH sits bedside, rubbing Eli's little arm as he lay
        asleep. NURSE VICKI peeks her head into the room.

                        NURSE VICKI
                Mrs. Logan, Eli's father is here.

        Sarah kisses Eli atop his head.

                        SARAH
                Mommy will be back shortly.

117   INT. UNIVERSITY OF COLORADO HOSPITAL- DAY

        In the Family Consultation Room, DR. MORAN sits at a table
        with SARAH and HENRY sitting on either side of him.

                        DR. MORAN
                    (remorseful)
                Mr. And Mrs. Logan, the x-rays are
                showing no improvement. I'm sorry.
                (beat) But we also have another
                concern. It appears that he has
                come down with PCP.

        Henry scowls.

                        HENRY
                You're going to have to speak in
                English, Doc.

                        DR. MORAN
                Pardon me, Mr. Logan. PCP is a type
                of pneumonia that is caused by a
                yeast-like fungus. It can often
                appear in patients with a weakened
                immune system. (beat) I've asked
                you both to join me today to
                discuss... well, what your decision
                would be should Eli code.

                        SARAH
                    (to Henry)
                Should his heart stop beating.

                        HENRY
                I know what it means. So... what,
                are you two wanting to pull the
                plug on my son?

                  DR. MORAN
        Mr. Logan--

                  SARAH
        Henry, we need to be on the same
        page when--

                  HENRY
        When, what? My son dies?

Henry springs to his feet, kicking his chair over backwards.

                  HENRY (CONT'D)
        I'm not talking about this. And I'm
        not gonna pull the plug on my son.

Henry bolts out of the room.

118   INT. UNIVERSITY OF COLORADO HOSPITAL- NIGHT

SARAH and ANNA sit in a quiet, dimly lit hospital room,
watching over a sleeping Eli. Sarah is holding Eli's hand.

                  SARAH
        I'll never understand.

                  ANNA
        What's that?

                  SARAH
        Why so many children have to go
        through so much pain.

                  ANNA
        Isn't it amazing how, when we were
        young, life was just all about us-
        when the most important part of our
        day as a teenager was trying to
        impress some guy?

Sarah smirks, accusingly.

                  SARAH
        Like Jimmy Nolan?

                  ANNA
        I was thinking more like Charlie
        Perkins.

They quietly chuckle.

                    SARAH
          Oh goodness... what were we
          thinking?

                    ANNA
          Right? (beat) But in the midst of
          our darkest hour, God sends us a
          little angel... and everything we
          have ever believed to be important
          just--

                    SARAH
          Vanishes.

                    ANNA
          It's almost like it's God's way of
          saving us from ourselves.

While staring intently at Eli, Sarah has a moment of clarity.

                    SARAH
               (to herself)
          By sending us an angel...

                    ANNA
          What was that?

                    SARAH
          An angel... a ministering spirit.
          Sent to save us from ourselves.

Sarah springs to her feet, looking at Eli.

                    ANNA
          What is it?

                    SARAH
          He stopped breathing.

Sarah grabs him by the shoulders, shaking him.

                    SARAH (CONT'D)
          Eli. Eli, baby.

Nothing. Sarah punches the call button, then shakes him
again.

He finally takes a deep breath. The RESPIRATORY THERAPIST, an
average height female (40S), along with other nurses rush
into the room. Sarah motions for them to freeze.

> SARAH (CONT'D)
> He'd stopped breathing for about
> twenty seconds, but now he's
> breathing again.

Everyone quietly and anxiously awaits. Watching. Eli.
Breathing.

He stops breathing again. The nurses jump into action.

> RESPIRATORY THERAPIST
> Mrs. Logan, I'm the respiratory
> therapist on duty.
>   (to nurses)
> ICU. Stat.

The nurses prepare to wheel Eli to ICU.

> SARAH
> I'm not leaving my son.

Briefly resisting, the Respiratory therapist gives in.

> RESPIRATORY THERAPIST
>   (to Sarah)
> Can you bag him?

> SARAH
> Yes.

> RESPIRATORY THERAPIST
>   (to nurses)
> I said, now.

Sarah places the oxygen bag over Eli's nose and mouth as they
wheel the gurney out of the room.

119   INT. UNIVERSITY OF COLORADO HOSPITAL- LATER

As the nurses bust into the ICU with Eli on the gurney, and
SARAH pumping the oxygen bag, the RESPIRATORY THERAPIST grabs
Sarah.

> RESPIRATORY THERAPIST
> Mrs. Logan, we'll take it from
> here.

> SARAH
> I said I'm not leaving my son.

Anna grabs Sarah, slowing her momentum at the door.

102

> RESPIRATORY THERAPIST
> Mrs. Logan, let us do our job.

> SARAH
> Do what you have to do! But I'm not
> leaving my son!

The Respiratory Therapist is perturbed.

> RESPIRATORY THERAPIST
> Well stay out of the way.

Sarah stands at the foot of the bed, watching as Eli is
intubated twice. With blood gushing, one of the nurses
quickly pushes in 60mls of IV platelets.

120   INT. UNIVERSITY OF COLORADO HOSPITAL- LATER

SARAH and Anna are in the ICU waiting room. SARAH is
nerveracking-ly pacing a hole in the floor.

> SARAH
> I wish someone would tell us
> something.

She shouts toward the ladies at the ICU nurses station...

> SARAH (CONT'D)
> Anything.

Anna sits calmly in a chair.

The ICU hallway doors open. DR. MORAN walks through,
approaching Sarah.

> SARAH (CONT'D)
> How is he?

> DR. MORAN
> He's stable for the time being. It
> appears his airway was being
> blocked by a swollen epiglottis,
> which can be a common side effect
> from the treatments that he's had
> to undergo.

Sarah thanks the Doctor while rushing to see Eli.

121   UNIVERSITY OF COLORADO HOSPITAL- DAY

SUPERIMPOSE:
> ICU - October 2nd, 1990

Eli is hooked up to numerous different tubes.

Nurse Vicki finishes administering Eli's drip, as SARAH
stands next to DR. MORAN in the doorway of the room.

> SARAH
> Okay, so what does this mean?

> DR. MORAN
> Along with his antibiotics and
> vitamins, we've also administered
> Pavalon, which will ensure that he
> won't panic and begin pulling on
> the tubes.

> SARAH
> So he can't move, but can he still
> hear me?

> DR. MORAN
> Absolutely Mrs. Logan. Just go
> about being the same, wonderful
> mother you are.

> SARAH
> Thank you Doctor.

> DR. MORAN
> I'll check back in soon, Sarah.

As the doctor and Nurse Vicki exit the room, Sarah takes a
deep breath before settling closely to Eli- left bedside.

Taking Eli by the hand, she leans in for a kiss, lays her
head beside his chest, and drapes her arm over his tiny,
frail body.

A solitaire tear rolls down the cheek of Eli.

> FADE OUT.

122   UNIVERSITY OF COLORADO HOSPITAL- DAY

SUPERIMPOSE:
> October 6th, 1990

With eyes closed, Eli lay motionless on the bed in PICU,
SARAH performs Range of Motion exercises.

She has his left leg suspended in the air bending it back and
forth at the knee while counting.

                    SARAH
          Seven, and eight, and nine, and
          ten... and one to grow on.

Sarah rests Eli's left leg back down onto the bed.

                    SARAH (CONT'D)
          Okay. Now I'm going to turn you
          onto your side so I can wash your
          back, honey.

Sarah reaches over, pulls a drenched cloth from a wash pan
and wrings it out. She then rolls Eli onto his side and
begins washing his back.

                    SARAH (CONT'D)
          Nurse Vicki called.

She leans down, kissing Eli on the back.

                    SARAH (CONT'D)
          She said she's got a new haircut
          that she can't wait to show you.
          And Hannah said to tell you hello
          and that she loves you. And Noah...

Sarah pauses, getting teary-eyed.

                    SARAH (CONT'D)
          ...Big brother just can't wait to
          see you again.

Sarah's hand slowly stops moving to and fro over Eli's back,
as she cuddles up to him from behind and rests her chin upon
the back of his shoulder.

                    SARAH (CONT'D)
          And mommy wants to tell you
          something, love.

She gently begins rubbing his arm...

                    SARAH (CONT'D)
          I wanted to tell you that I'm so
          proud of you, and that I love you
          so much. A while back when you woke
          up in the middle of the night
          wanting watermelon, I drove through
          half of Denver to find it for you -
          because I love you so much.
                    (MORE)

                    SARAH (CONT'D)
And I'd eat mountains and mountains
of green peas, Eli, if that would
make you all better- because I love
you so much. But what I really
wanted to tell you, Eli...

Sarah begins crying.

                    SARAH (CONT'D)
...Is that mommy's sorry. I'm sorry
I haven't been able to fix you all
better. And if you want to go to
Heaven and Jesus, well that's
alright with mommy.

Sarah squeezes Eli tightly. Motionless, with eyes still
closed, a tear rolls down his cheek.

123   UNIVERSITY OF COLORADO HOSPITAL- DAY

SUPERIMPOSE:
               October 9th, 1990

In the Family Consultation Room, SARAH and HENRY sit across
the desk from DR. MORAN.

                    DR. MORAN
We've done as you've requested Mrs.
Logan, and have added the ice
blankets in order to help with his
fever spikes.

                    SARAH
Thank you, Doctor.

                    DR. MORAN
Now, the latest x-rays, I'm sorry
to say, show no signs of
improvement on his lungs. And we're
still trying to determine what it
is that continues to insult his
liver.

                    HENRY
So what does all of that mean?

                    DR. MORAN
It means we can do one of two
things, Mr. Logan.
               (MORE)

                    DR. MORAN (CONT'D)
          We can either continue with our
          current treatments, which means
          we'd keep him as comfortable as
          possible while continually
          increasing his pressure settings on
          the ventilator. Or, we can perform
          a lung biopsy with the hopes of
          determining exactly what is
          infecting his lungs.

                    SARAH
          But would a biopsy be safe?

                    DR. MORAN
          To be honest, Sarah, if we
          performed the biopsy, we'd be
          running the risk of losing him
          right there on the operating table.

                    HENRY
          Then let's just keep doing what
          we're doing till he gets better.

Sarah shakes her head, sighs, and springs to her feet.

                    SARAH
          Don't you get it, Henry!? Eli's not
          getting better!

Henry's pride turns to a look of helplessness, as he
stutters...

                    HENRY
          Th... Then what are we supposed to
          do, Sarah?

Sarah just shakes her head and makes her way to the door, as
Henry begs of her...

                    HENRY (CONT'D)
          Sarah, what are we supposed to do?

Opening the office door, she peeks back over her shoulder...

                    SARAH
          You're such a coward, Henry.

She leaves, closing the door behind her.

124   HALLWAY

Sarah's lip quivers as she approaches the nurses station.

                    SARAH
          Can I borrow a phone please?

Noticing Sarah's state of despair, the OLD NURSE #2 (70's),
and petite, spins the phone around.

                    OLD NURSE #2
          Why sure, dear.

Sarah quickly dials a number.

                    NOAH (V.O.)
          Hello?

Sarah fights the explosion of tears when hearing Noah's
voice.

INTERCUT SARAH/NOAH

                    SARAH
               (into phone)
          Hey Noah, it's mommy.

                    NOAH (V.O.)
          Mommy, I got to ride on a fire
          truck today! I even got a fireman's
          hat.

Sarah places her hand over her mouth, trying to maintain her
composure.

                    SARAH
               (into phone)
          Really...?

                    NOAH (V.O.)
          Yeah! But I forgot to get one for
          Eli--

Sarah begins to break.

                    SARAH
          That's great. I'll give you a call
          back a little later, Noah. Mommy
          loves you.

                    NOAH
          Love you too Mommy, and Eli.

                    SARAH
          Okay. Bye...

Sarah hangs up the phone. Sliding down the front of the
nurses station to the floor, she bitterly weeps.

125   UNIVERSITY OF COLORADO HOSPITAL- DAY

SUPERIMPOSE:
                    October 15th, 1990
                        11:00am

DR. MORAN and SARAH sit in the Family Consultation room,
waiting, as HENRY finally makes a late entrance.

Dr. Moran begins once Henry has taken his seat.

                    DR. MORAN
          Henry. Sarah. There never is an
          easy way to have a conversation
          such as this. But we must do so
          nonetheless. (beat). At this time,
          we can continue with the current
          treatment, and Eli might be able to
          hang on for one more day.

The doctor takes a brief pause, allowing Sarah and Henry to
absorb what has been said, as numbness sets in with them
both.

                    DR. MORAN (CONT'D)
          A second option would be to slowly
          decrease the ventilator settings,
          weaning him off until... he takes
          his last breath. Or a third option-
          and this because that little guy is
          so tough and has a heart that
          refuses to give out- we can give
          that germ inside him hell, in one
          last effort to save him and keep
          him alive.

                    HENRY
          Let's do it.

                    SARAH
          Wait a minute. I understand what
          you're saying Dr. Moran, but I
          don't want my son to be in anymore
          pain.

                    HENRY
          So what are you saying, that we
          should just give up?

Sarah looks at Dr. Moran with confidence.

                    SARAH
          No.

126   UNIVERSITY OF COLORADO HOSPITAL- DAY

SUPERIMPOSE:
                    2:21PM

DR. MORAN, SARAH and HENRY stand at Eli's bedside- SARAH on
one side, HENRY and the doctor on the other. Nurse Vicki
stands off to the side.

                    DR. MORAN
                 (to Sarah)
            He should be waking up any time
            now.

Sarah leans down, softly stroking Eli's cheek with the back
of her fingers.

                    SARAH
            Eli. Eli, honey. It's mommy.

No response.

Sarah then leans over, kissing him on the brow.

                    SARAH (CONT'D)
            Eli, honey. It's mommy.

Eli opens his eyes. Henry steps in closer.

                    HENRY
            Hey buddy. Your daddy's here too.

Sarah peers deep into Eli's eyes.

                    SARAH
            Eli, we wanted to ask you if it
            would be okay to try a lot of new
            medicine to try and kill the rest
            of these cancer ghosts. If you want
            us to, then open your eyes real big
            for mommy. But only if you want to
            try one more time.

In a moment in time that seems to last forever, with what
little strength he has left, Eli musters the courage to open
his eyes wide.

Sarah is overcome with emotion and sprays him with kisses.

                    SARAH (CONT'D)
            Mommy and Daddy are so proud of you
            son. You're the strongest little
            boy in the world.

127   UNIVERSITY OF COLORADO HOSPITAL- DAY

        SUPERIMPOSE:
                        3:13PM

        Nurse Vicki administers the new medicine into the drip.
        Sarah, DR. MORAN, Nurse Vicki and Henry all watch with great
        anticipation.

        While leaving, Dr. Moran pauses at Sarah's side.

                        DR. MORAN
                Only time will tell.

128   UNIVERSITY OF COLORADO HOSPITAL- NIGHT

        SUPERIMPOSE:
                        5:20PM

        Sarah sits bedside, tightly clinging to Eli. Henry paces the
        floor as Nurse Vicki checks on Eli.

129   UNIVERSITY OF COLORADO HOSPITAL- LATER

        Sarah sits bedside, alone in the room, tightly clinging to
        Eli. She looks to the clock on the wall that reads...

        ONSCREEN: 7:27PM

130   UNIVERSITY OF COLORADO HOSPITAL- LATER

        Sarah, bedside, clasps her hands around one of Eli's. Kissing
        his hand, she then loving grins and pets his cheek.

        Henry sits in a chair in a back corner of the room, flipping
        pages of a magazine.

131   UNIVERSITY OF COLORADO HOSPITAL- LATER

        SUPERIMPOSE:
                        11:19PM

        SARAH, bedside, clinging to Eli, awaits patiently for him to
        respond to the new dose of meds. The heart monitor beeps.

        Looking over, SARAH finds HENRY asleep in the chair in the
        corner of the room. The heart monitor beeps.

Sarah's focus comes back to Eli, and his precious little
face. The heart monitor somewhat slows, grabbing Sarah's
attention.

Sarah stands to check on the monitor.

The beeping stops...

Sarah punches the call button! Nurse Vicki and DR. MORAN
storm through the door shortly thereafter.

Sarah in a panic...

>   SARAH
>   (to Dr. Moran)
>   It just stopped beating!

Henry leaps from the chair to the scene...

>   HENRY
>   What's happening? What's going on?

Dr. Moran looks to Henry and Sarah for approval...

>   DR. MORAN
>   His heart has stopped.

Henry points to Eli's chest - compressing up and down...

>   HENRY
>   Then how's he still breathing

>   DR. MORAN
>   That's from the ventilator.

>   HENRY
>   Well do something!

Nurse Vicki pulls out a syringe, jabbing it into the IV.

Everyone pauses as the room becomes eerie quiet.

The heart monitor finally begins to slowly beep.

Sarah quickly plants her head next to Eli's.

>   SARAH
>   I love you so much, Eli. Mommy's
>   here, and I'm not going anywhere. I
>   love you my son.

>   HENRY
>   (to Dr. Moran)
>   Now what?

                    DR. MORAN
          Mr. Logan, There's no guarantees--

The heart monitor stops beeping.

Sarah wails and weeps bitterly.

                    HENRY
          Give the heart medicine again, now!

Nurse Vicki looks to Dr. Moran as he gives her a shameful nod
to proceed.

Nurse Vicki grabs another syringe and jabs it into the IV.

Sarah is gripped tightly to Eli.

                    SARAH
          No Henry! Stop it!

Nurse Vicki administers the meds. The room is still, as only
Sarah's weeping can be heard.

Sarah has a limp Eli pulled into her bosom, showering him
with kisses and words of love.

Beep. Beep. The heart monitor begins to chime again.

Henry begins yelling at Dr. Moran and Nurse Vicki.

Slowly laying Eli's tiny head back down, Sarah notices an
object protruding from beneath his pillow.

Henry's bickering with the doctor becomes like a faint
whisper in the background as Sarah enters into a moment of
serenity. She pulls the object from beneath the pillow and
into the light.

Wiping away the tears, she is able to focus on the object in
her hand.

ONSCREEN: It is a tiny, wooden angel that reads, JOSHUA.

With faint echoes of Henry's bickering in the b.g., Sarah is
solely focused upon Eli.

Slowly leaning down and resting her cheek near his, she
whispers into Eli's hear...

                    SARAH (CONT'D)
          It's okay. It's okay to fly away.
          Mommy will be with you soon. I love
          you. I love you!

Sarah's moment of serenity is diminished as Henry's bickering comes to an abrupt halt, brought on by a singular, continuous beep coming from the heart monitor.

>   HENRY
>   Do it again!

Sarah, wailing once more, pulls her son into her bosom and cries out at Henry.

>   SARAH
>   Henry! No more, Henry! Let him go!
>   Let my son go...

Dr. Moran motions to Nurse Vicki to "wait."

Henry looks to Sarah. After a beat, his look of anger turns to one of downcast, and his tensed shoulders begin to release in a slouch. Finally giving a slight nod of agreement, Henry slowly falls back against the wall and slides down to the floor.

Sarah showers her little boy with tear-filled mommy kisses.

>   MATCH CUT TO:

132   UNIVERSITY OF COLORADO HOSPITAL- LATER

Dr. Moran and Nurse Vicki disappear, as Henry still sits in the floor with his face buried in his hands.

SARAH sits in a chair rocking a lifeless Eli.

>   SARAH (V.O.)
>   On October 15th, 1990, at 11:35pm,
>   my little boy went to Heaven and
>   Jesus. Just like he had been
>   wanting to do.

>   MATCH CUT TO:

133   EXT. SARAH LOGAN'S HOUSE- DAY 2016

We see the hands of a fifty-six-year-old woman. One hand is writing in a journal that rests in her lap, while the other holds tightly to a Kleenex tissue. A wool sweater blankets her arms down to the wrists.

>   SARAH (V.O.)
>   We buried little Eli on October
>   18th, 1990.

From the front yard, we see a fifty-six-year-old Sarah Logan
sitting in a rocking chair on her shaded front porch, writing
in her journal.

> SARAH (V.O.)
> I've been asked on several
> occasions following that day, if
> life gets any better after having
> lost a child.

Sarah briefly looks up and across the front yard, intently
thinking, before putting pen back to paper.

> SARAH (V.O.)
> I guess my answer would have to be,
> "Sometimes." There are definitely
> those days when I feel so much joy
> inside, knowing that my little Eli
> is in Heaven. I must confess,
> however, it took me twenty-three
> years to accept and receive that
> joy; and a little less time with
> Joshua.

Sarah pauses, places her pen inside the journal and closes it
shut, placing it on the end table beside her. From afar, we
see Sarah once again staring intently out across the front
yard, as the focus on her face begins to slowly draw nearer
and nearer.

> SARAH (V.O.)
> But through it all, what I've
> discovered most is that life on
> earth... for all of us really, is
> not a fairy-tale, but rather a
> restless journey. For, no matter
> which path you choose, each will
> lead you to "The Land of
> Paradox..."

The focus continues to draw closer and closer to Sarah.

> SARAH
> ...Where you'll find the best and
> worst that this life has to offer.
> You'll find both joy and pain,
> happiness and sorrow, love and
> hatred. (beat) And unlike
> Cinderella, it wasn't a prince that
> I found in "The Land of Paradox,"
> rather, it was two kings. The One I
> call my Lord and Savior. And the
> other...

The focus of the camera finally comes to a stop on a close-up of Sarah's face.

> SARAH (V.O.)
> ...The King of Loss.

FADE OUT.

134   ROLL CREDITS

NARRATIVE BIOGRAPHY

MARY SCHMIDT & JOSHUA VICKERY

Mary Schmidt is a retired Registered Nurse. However, being retired most definitely does not mean that she is inactive.

Having grown up in central Kansas, both Mary and her husband, Michael, greatly enjoy finding the time to frequent the mountains of Colorado. They both enjoy traveling, reading together, playing poker, and off road 4-wheeling in the mountains.

Back at home, both Mary and Michael are active members of the Catholic Church, where Mary has taught Kindergarten Catechism. She has also worked in various capacities for the American Cancer Society, March of Dimes, and both the Boy and Cub Scouts (where her son, Gene, is an Eagle Scout). She and her husband have also had the wonderful opportunity of sponsoring trips for high school music students.

Mary absolutely loves all forms of art, but mostly focuses on the visual arts such as amateur photography, along with traditional and graphic art as her disabilities allow.

Joshua Vickery is a professional Christian freelance writer of novels and screenplays. However, he spends a majority of his time now as a Christian copywriter, helping to grown Christian businesses and ministries.

As a young man, he was gifted to enjoy the opportunity of playing college baseball. After college, he then traveled much of the Mid-Western United States as a Country Music singer. However, having been raised in the foothills of the Ozark Mountains, his love for family has him settled back home in Northwest Arkansas.

Having married the woman of his dreams, Christina, in 2003, he was then able to adopt her daughter shortly thereafter. Joshua and Christina have recently had the wonderful privilege of watching their daughter, Madison, graduate from high school and begin her first year of college. However, Joshua received another wonderful gift in 2009 when his wife gave birth to their now, seven-year-old son, Cross.

His life mission is that of Christian love, where he defines it as an action or series of actions that cause intrinsic value in others.